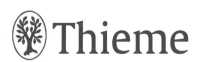

Burghardt's Primary Care Colposcopy

Textbook and Atlas

Olaf Reich, MD
Associate Professor of Gynecology
Associate Professor of Patholgy
Department of Obstetrics and Gynecology
Medical University of Graz
Graz, Austria

Frank Girardi, MD
Professor Emeritus
Department of Obstetrics and Gynecology
Medical University of Graz
Graz, Austria

Karl Tamussino, MD, FACS
Professor
Department of Obstetrics and Gynecology
Medical University of Graz
Graz, Austria

Hellmuth Pickel, MD
Professor Emeritus
Department of Obstetrics and Gynecology
Medical University of Graz
Graz, Austria

369 illustrations

Thieme
Stuttgart · New York · Delhi · Rio de Janerio

Library of Congress Cataloging-in-Publication Data is available from the publisher

This book represents selections from Girardi F., Reich O., Tamussino K., Pickel H. Burghardt's Colposcopy and Cervical Pathology, newly edited, published and copyrighted by Georg Thieme Verlag, Stuttgart, Germany 2015.

Important Note: Medicine is an ever-changing science undergoing continual development. Research and clinical experience are continually expanding our knowledge, in particular our knowledge of proper treatment and drug therapy. Insofar as this book mentions any dosage or application, readers may rest assured that the authors, editors, and publishers have made every effort to ensure that such references are in accordance with **the state of knowledge at the time of production of the book.**

Nevertheless, this does not involve, imply, or express any guarantee or responsibility on the part of the publishers with respect of any dosage instructions and forms of application stated in the book. **Every user is requested to examine carefully** the manufacturer's leaflets accompanying each drug and to check, if necessary in consultation with a physician or specialist, whether the dosage schedules mentioned therein or the contraindications stated by the manufacturer differ from the statements made in the present book. Such examination is particularly important with drugs that are either rarely used or have been newly released on the market. Every dosage schedule or every form of application used is entirely at the user's risk and responsibility. The authors and publishers request every user to report to the publishers any discrepancies or inaccuracies noticed.

Some of the product names, patents, and registered designs referred to in this book are in fact registered trademarks or proprietary names, even though specific reference to this fact is not always made in the text. Therefore, the appearance of a name without a designation as proprietary is not to be construed as a representation by the publisher that it is in the public domain.

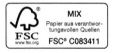

© 2017 by Georg Thieme Verlag KG

Thieme Publishers Stuttgart
Rüdigerstrasse 14, 70469 Stuttgart, Germany
+49 [0]711 8931 421, customerservice@thieme.de

Thieme Publishers New York
333 Seventh Avenue, New York, NY 10001 USA
+1 800 782 3488, customerservice@thieme.com

Thieme Publishers Delhi
A-12, Second Floor, Sector-2, Noida-201301
Uttar Pradesh, India
+91 120 45 566 00, customerservice@thieme.in

Thieme Publishers Rio, Thieme Publicações Ltda.
Edifício Rodolpho de Paoli, 25º andar
Av. Nilo Peçanha, 50 - Sala 2508
Rio de Janeiro 20020-906 Brasil
+55 21 3172 2297 / +55 21 3172 1896

Cover design: Thieme Publishing Group
Typesetting by DiTech Process Solutions, India

Printed in Germany by CPI Books GmbH   5 4 3 2 1

ISBN 978-3-13-130722-4

Also available as an e-book:
eISBN 978-3-13-162712-4

Contents

Contents

Preface

Colposcopy is a widely used technique to visually examine the lower genital tract with exposure, a light source, and magnification. The number of textbooks on colposcopy testifies to the rapid development of the technique over the last 20 years. The first edition of the full version of this book was published in German in 1984. Since then revised editions of the full version, now called *Burghardt's Colposcopy and Cervical Pathology* in honor of Erich Burghardt who passed away in 2006, have appeared in Spanish, Japanese, French, Italian, and English. The present edition of the compact edition is user-oriented resource for general practitioners, nurses, and other nonspecialists. Accordingly, we have left out detailed histologic pictures and descriptions while keeping the colposcopic images that are the backbone of the book. So-called "extended colposcopy" (i.e., with the acetic acid and the iodine test) is given ample coverage. Like its predecessors, this book intends to explain both the fundamentals of colposcopic technique and how colposcopy can help one appreciate the dynamic processes at the cervix and lower genital tract that we have to understand to prevent invasive cervical cancer and neoplasias of the vulva, vagina, and anus.

We thank Dr. Charles Redman (Stoke on Trent) and Dr. Esther Moss (Leicester) for their contribution to the chapter Teaching Colposcopy.

We would like to thank Thieme Verlag for their longstanding support of this project. And, of course, we thank our wives—Christine, Ursula, Caroline, and Ulrike—for their support.

Olaf Reich,
Frank Girardi,
Karl Tamussino,
Hellmuth Pickel

Chapter 1

Human Papillomaviruses and Cervical Cancer

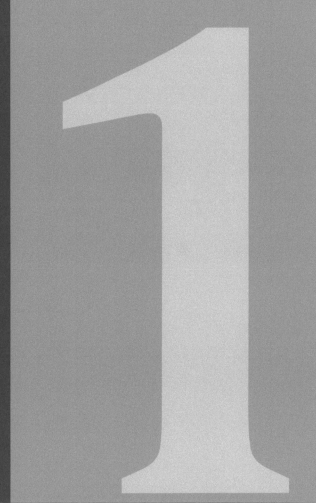

1 Human Papillomaviruses and Cervical Cancer

During much of the 20th century, cervical cancer was a scourge. In large parts of the world, this remains the case, the disease often striking women younger than 40 years. In 1908, Friedrich Schauta in Vienna ended his monograph on radical vaginal hysterectomy for cervical cancer on the note that "the early detection of uterine cancer is the greatest challenge facing future generations of academic teachers and practicing physicians." In the same year, Howard Kelly in Baltimore wrote that "the only avenue open with certainty to progress today lies in the direction of discovering our cases of cancer at an earlier stage in the disease." Physicians battling this disease appreciated the importance of early detection, but did not know how to get there.

1.1 Etiology of Cervical Cancer

Papillomaviruses are a large and diverse group of small DNA viruses that infect epithelial tissues, and have evolved over millions of years. As parasites, they use species-specific animals and humans for replication. About 120 types of cutaneous or mucosal human papillomavirus (HPV) have been described in humans.

HPVs have a simple structure and are built of only a few proteins. The small circular genomes are organized into a set of six early genes (*E6, E7, E1, E2, E4,* and *E5*), which are involved in viral gene expression and replication control, and two late genes (*L1* and *L2*), which encode the major capsid proteins. In cervical carcinogenesis, two of the early genes (*E6* and *E7*) can transform cervical epithelium.

In 1976, Harald zur Hausen found the DNA of HPVs in cervical cancers and genital warts. In 1983, investigators in zur Hausen's laboratory established HPV 16 as the leading candidate in the etiology of preinvasive and invasive cervical neoplasia. HPV types are widely classified into low-risk and high-risk groups according to their ability to promote malignant transformation. HPV types 16, 18, 31, 33, and others are now classified as high-risk types. In contrast, HPV 6, 11, 40, 42, and others are rarely found in cervical cancer and are considered low-risk types.

All cervical epithelia are vulnerable to HPV infection. The development of cervical cancer and its precursor lesions requires persisting infection with high-risk HPV (HR-HPV). HPV 16 infection results in predominantly squamous neoplasia, whereas HPV 18 and 45 have a greater tendency to induce glandular neoplasia. HPV 16 and 18 cause about 70% of cervical cancers. Together with HPV 31 and 45, and cofactors (e.g., smoking, immunodeficiency, number of sexual partners), they are the prime risk factors for cervical cancer.

Worldwide, about 300 million women are infected with HPVs. The majority of genital HPV infections remain asymptomatic, and the majority of infections resolve spontaneously. Genital HPV infection is transmitted almost exclusively through sexual and genital skin-to-skin contact. Most women acquire cervical HPV infection within a few years of initiating sexual intercourse. Coinfection with more than one HPV genotype is common, especially in young women. Most HPV infections clear as a result of cell-mediated immune response. About 90% of women with HPV infection become HPV-negative within 2 years. The peak rate of HPV infection is seen in women younger than 25 years, with a decline that plateaus around 30 to 35 years. In some countries, there is a slight increase in women over 50 years.

1.2 Natural History of Cervical Cancer

HPVs infect epithelial basal cells (reserve cells), which are responsible for regeneration of the epithelium (Fig. 1.1). Subcolumnar reserve cells enable metaplasia from columnar to squamous epithelium.

HPV infection probably occurs when minor trauma (e.g., sexual intercourse) exposes the basal cells (reserve cells) of the cervical mucosa to the virus. Expression of viral genes in individual infected basal cells leads to lateral extension of the initially HPV-infected cell clone (Fig. 1.2a,b).

The time from HPV infection to the development of high-grade squamous intraepithelial lesions (HSIL) varies widely. Generally, persisting infection with HPV 16, 18, or 45 entails a 20 to 30% risk for cervical intraepithelial neoplasia grade III (CIN 3, HSIL) over the next 5 years. However, some high-grade lesions, particularly with HPV 16 infection, develop quickly (i.e., 1 or 2 years after infection). Women with multiple HR-HPV infections are at increased risk.

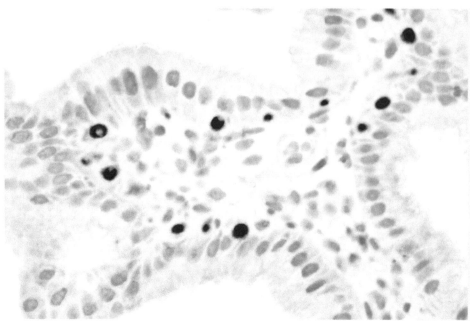

Fig. 1.1 Individual reserve cells in the basal layer of the columnar epithelium. The nuclei stain darkly for p63.

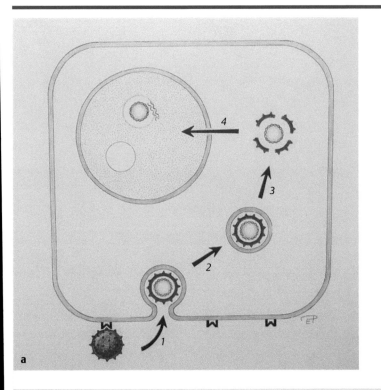

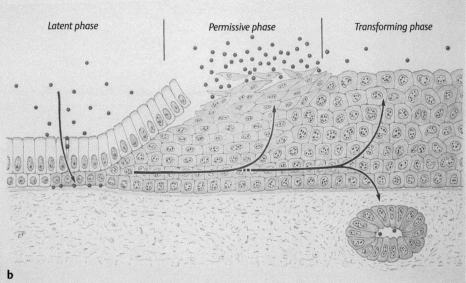

Latent phase | Permissive phase | Transforming phase

Fig.1.2 (a) HPV entry model: uptake of HPV into the basal cells is mediated by endocytosis. Upon release from the particle, the circular viral genome is transported to the nucleus, where it resides as an extrachromosomal molecule. **(b)** Schematic description of the three distinct phases of HPV infection at the cervix. Minor lacerations of the epithelium permits contact of HPV with the cervical reserve (basal) cells. In the latent phase, the HPV genome releases viral copies in low numbers and without significant viral gene expression. In some instances, low levels of viral gene expression occur and result in viral replication (permissive phase). The late gene products permit packaging of the replicated viral genomes, and newly produced HPVs are released at the surface of the cervix. Morphologic effects include low-grade squamous intraepithelial lesions (LSIL). Transforming infections cause HSIL and adenocarcinoma in situ (AIS).

Cervical cancer is an occasional and late manifestation of infection with HR-HPV. The latency from initial HPV infection to invasive cancer is in the range of 8 years and more. HSIL correlates with a greater risk of progression to invasion than low-grade squamous intraepithelial lesions (LSIL). Spontaneous regression can occur in about 57, 43, and 32% of cases of CIN 1, CIN 2, and CIN 3 lesions, respectively, and persistence in 32, 35, and 56%. Only about 1% of CIN 1 lesions and 5% of CIN 2 lesions but more than 12% of CIN 3 lesions progress to invasive cervical cancer. In one study, untreated CIN 3 had a 30% probability of becoming invasive over a 30-year period.

1.2.1 Phases of HPV Infection

HPV infections go through three phases of viral gene expression: the latent phase, the permissive (productive) phase, and the transforming phase. After intraepithelial neoplastic transformation, some HSIL and adenocarcinoma in situ (AIS) will progress to invasive cervical cancer (Fig. 1.2).

Latent Phase

Latent infection does not produce infectious particles, remains clinically inapparent, and triggers no histopathologic changes. Most HPV infections probably end this way, without initiation of major viral gene expression.

Permissive (Productive) Phase

Permissive (productive) infection shows no signs of cellular transformation and can be caused by either low-risk or high-risk HPV types. It frequently results in characteristic morphologic changes of the infected cervical squamous epithelium (koilocytosis) (Fig. 1.3). This corresponds to condylomas or CIN 1 in histologic specimens or LSIL in cytologic specimens. Probably about 90% of productive infections become undetectable within 1 to 2 years, corresponding to spontaneous resolution of LSIL.

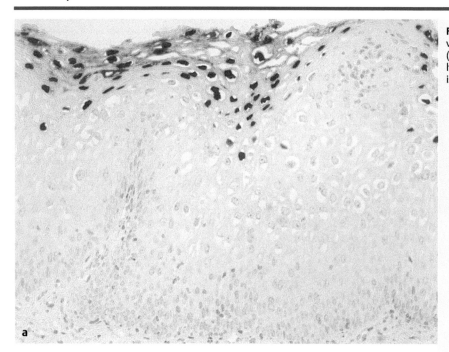

Fig. 1.3 (a, b) Permissive (productive) HPV infection with viral replication. **(a)** Staining for L1 shows HPV capsid protein (red) in superficial layers of the infected epithelium. **(b)** In situ hybridization shows newly produced HPVs (blue). (This image is provided courtesy of S. Syrjänen.)

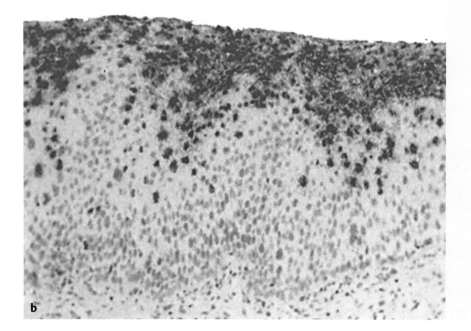

Transforming Phase

Transforming infections are almost always associated with HR-HPV types. Transforming infections cause high-grade lesions. These lesions are referred to as CIN 2/3 in histology and HSIL in cytologic specimens (Fig. 1.4). For cancer to develop, HPV has to evade immune detection over a prolonged period for genetic abnormalities to accumulate. Not all HSIL or AIS will progress to invasive cancer.

1.3 Morphogenesis of Cervical Cancer

Squamous cell cervical cancer can develop in metaplastic squamous epithelium (inside the transformation zone) or in the original squamous epithelium.

1.3.1 Morphogenesis of Squamous Cell Carcinoma in Metaplastic Epithelium

Squamous cell carcinoma inside the transformation zone develops via SIL in fields of squamous epithelium of metaplastic origin. Metaplasia begins with the appearance of a row of subcolumnar reserve cells in a well-defined field (Figs. 1.5a–c and 1.6a–d). Later, immature metaplastic squamous epithelium can become mature (Fig. 1.7). Different fields of (immature and mature) metaplastic squamous epithelium can arise on the same cervix, simultaneously or at different times. If present, HPV infection usually does not affect the entire metaplastic epithelium. In permissive (productive) infections, virus replication is also limited to sharply defined fields (Fig. 1.8).

HSIL can appear at the very beginning of the metaplastic process without LSIL. Atypical cells arise simultaneously from the

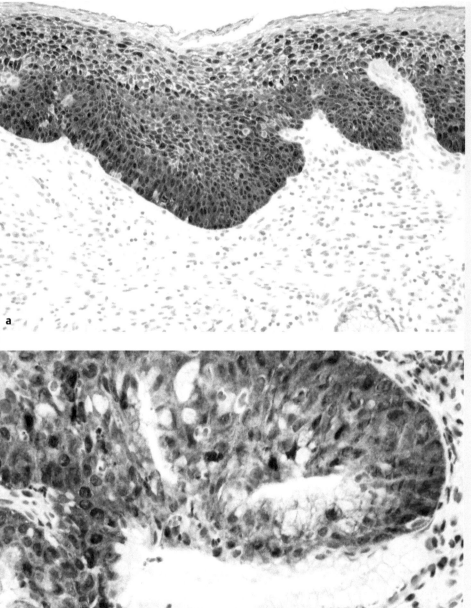

Fig. 1.4 (a, b) HSIL with diffuse overexpression of p16^{INK4a} in all cells of the proliferating compartment at the surface **(a)** and in a cervical crypt **(b)**. In the transforming phase of HPV infection, the early viral genes E6 and E7 are strongly expressed and p16^{INK4a} is upregulated and overexpressed.

base of whole fields of metaplastic epithelium, not from single cells in an initial focus (Fig. 1.9a,b).

Squamous metaplasia and SIL frequently coexist in separate fields on the same cervix. Adjacent fields are separated by sharp borders. When caused by different HPV types, the appearance of SIL can differ from field to field, but the borders are also sharp (Fig. 1.10). In these cases, the entire lesion is a mosaic of independent primary lesions. SIL remains within its original boundaries and does not enlarge by active surface spread. It grows, enlarges, and spreads by recruiting or apposing new fields of varying appearance.

The synchronous or metachronous development of SIL in various epithelial fields and its confluence play a central role in understanding the pathogenesis of cervical cancer because the likelihood of invasion increases with the surface area of a lesion, which is directly related to the total size. Invasion proceeds unifocally or multifocally from the base of larger lesions, with a small nest of cells penetrating the stroma, so-called early stromal invasion.

1.3.2 Morphogenesis of Squamous Cell Carcinoma in Original Squamous Epithelium

A small percentage of SILs develop in original squamous epithelium of the cervix, outside the TZ. This is not due to active spread of SIL toward the vagina across the original SCJ. SIL outside the TZ develops separately and arises by proliferation of the basal and parabasal layers of the original squamous epithelium.

1.3.3 Morphogenesis of Adenocarcinoma

Adenocarcinoma of the cervix develops via AIS, which is defined as noninvading but highly atypical columnar epithelium. There are no low-grade glandular lesions corresponding to LSIL. AISs most frequently arise at the TZ in fields, often in association with HSIL. As in SIL, the transition between the atypical and normal columnar epithelium is abrupt (Figs. 1.11 and 1.12). Both the

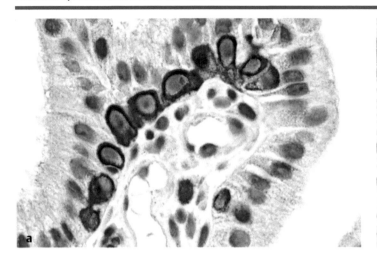
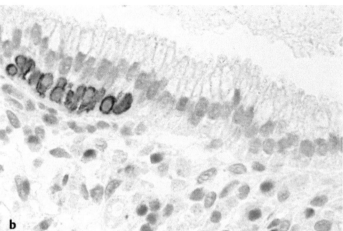
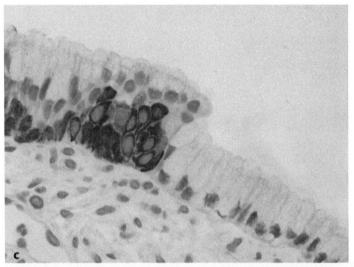

Fig. 1.5 (a–c) Rows of subcolumnar reserve cells as an early feature of squamous metaplasia of columnar epithelium **(a, b)**. Note the well-defined fields and the beginning proliferation of subcolumnar reserve cells **(c)** (staining for cytokeratin 17).

surface and the crypts can be involved by AIS. As in SIL, invasion of AIS proceeds from the base of the transformed epithelium, with a small nest of cells penetrating the stroma.

1.4 HPV Vaccines

The identification of HPVs as the causative agent of cervical cancer soon prompted research into the development of vaccines. Prophylactic vaccines were based on virus-like particles (VLPs) produced by expressing L1, the major capsid protein of HPV, using recombinant DNA technology. The VLPs preserve and resemble the structure of the native virus and induce antibodies cross-reactive with infectious virus particles. Antibodies reach high serum titers and reach the vaginal fluid by transudation.

Two vaccines, one quadrivalent and one bivalent, were developed and entered into clinical trials in 2001 and 2004, respectively. The FUTURE studies evaluated the efficacy of a prophylactic quadrivalent vaccine in preventing anogenital diseases associated with HPV types 6, 11, 16, and 18. Initially, a total of 5,455 women aged 16 to 24 years received the vaccine or a placebo and were evaluated for the incidence of genital warts,

vulvar or vaginal intraepithelial neoplasia (VIN/VAIN), or cancer and the incidence of CIN, AIS, or cancer associated with HPV type 6, 11, 16, or 18. In the primary analysis at 3 years of a per-protocol susceptible population of women who had no virologic evidence of HPV infection at baseline, vaccine efficacy for each of the coprimary end points was 100%, showing that the vaccine significantly reduced the incidence of HPV-associated anogenital diseases in young women. At 42 months' follow-up in the per-protocol susceptible population, the efficacy of the vaccine against lesions related to the HPV types in the vaccine was 96% for CIN 1, 100% for both VIN 1 and VAIN 1, and 99% for condylomata. In the FUTURE II study, a total of 12,167 women were randomized and evaluated for CIN 2/3, AIS, or cervical cancer related to HPV 16/18. After 3 years' follow-up, vaccine efficacy for the prevention of the primary composite end point in the per-protocol susceptible population was 99%.

The PApilloma TRIal against Cancer In young Adults (PATRICIA) included over 18,000 healthy women aged 15 to 25 years with no more than six lifetime sexual partners, irrespective of baseline HPV DNA status. Women were randomly assigned to receive a bivalent HPV 16/18 vaccine or a control hepatitis A vaccine. The primary end point was vaccine efficacy against CIN 2+ associated with HPV 16/18 in women who were seronegative at baseline.

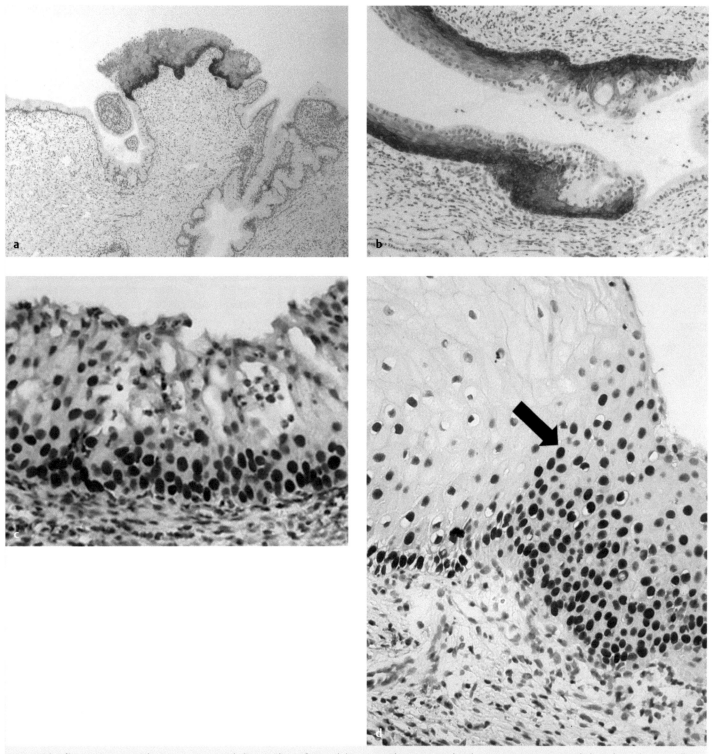

Fig. 1.6 (a–d) Immature metaplastic squamous epithelium at the surface and the crypts. The structure already suggests squamous epithelium, but columnar cells are still present (**a, b**: staining for cytokeratin 17). Note the proliferation of p63-positive subcolumnar reserve cells (**c**: staining for p63). (**d**) Sharp border between newly formed metaplastic squamous epithelium on the right and adjacent mature squamous epithelium on the left (**d**: staining for p63).

After a mean follow-up of 35 months, vaccine efficacy against CIN 2+ associated with HPV 16/18 was 93% in the primary analysis and 98% in an analysis of probable causality to HPV type in lesions with multiple oncogenic types. In the end-of-study analysis, vaccine efficacy was 93% against all CIN 3+ and 100% against CIN 3+ associated with HPV 16/18.

The quadrivalent vaccine (Gardasil, Merck & Co.) and the bivalent vaccine (Cervarix, GlaxoSmithKline Biologicals) were approved by the Food and Drug Administration in the United States in 2006 and 2009, respectively. HPV vaccines have been incorporated into vaccination programs and recommendations in many countries, including developing countries, where cervical cancer is a much larger public health problem. In 2015, results of a trial of a 9-valent vaccine (Gardasil 9, Merck & Co.) were published and this vaccine is becoming available worldwide.

The primary target population for HPV vaccination is adolescent girls before sexual debut. There is also substantial vaccine efficacy in a population approximating a general population of sexually active women, suggesting that catch-up vaccination will also provide benefit. Furthermore, women after surgical therapy of HPV-associated lesions (e.g., conization) after vaccination can continue to benefit from reduction in the risk of development of recurrent lesions. Both vaccines are generally less effective in immunocompromised individuals. Neither of the prophylactic vaccines has shown therapeutic activity.

PATRICIA and FUTURE were landmark studies. In 2007, Australia became one of the first countries to implement a nationally funded program for vaccination of girls and young women with the quadrivalent vaccine. An audit of national surveillance data through 2011 showed large declines in the proportions of young women diagnosed with genital warts in the vaccination period. Genital warts in heterosexual men also declined, probably as a result of herd immunity. These results indicate that HPV vaccines are highly effective outside the trial setting and strongly support their widespread implementation.

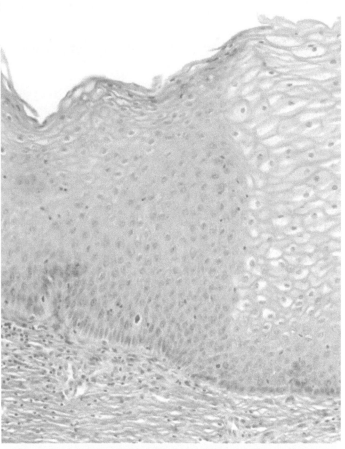

Fig. 1.7 Sharp border between mature metaplastic squamous epithelium on the left and normal squamous epithelium on the right hematoxylin and eosin.

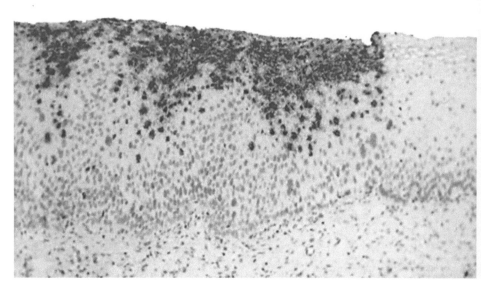

Fig. 1.8 Field of a permissive (productive) HPV infection of the squamous epithelium. Note the sharp border between the epithelium with viral replication on the left and the epithelium without HPV replication on the right (in situ hybridization). (This image is provided courtesy of S. Syrjänen.)

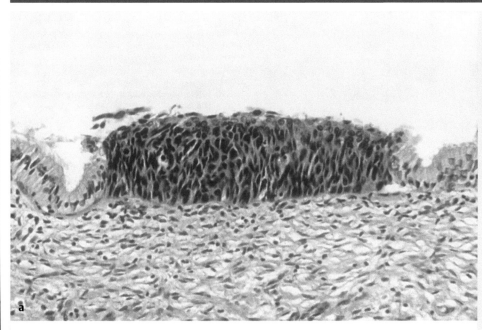

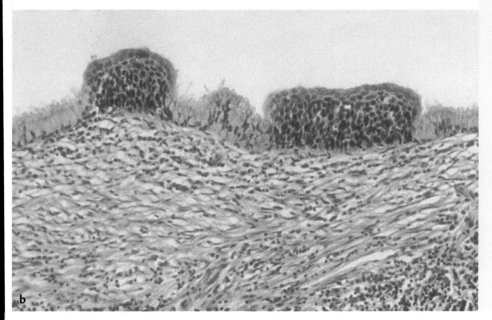

Fig. 1.9 High-grade squamous intraepithelial lesion at the beginning of the metaplastic process.
(a) Atypical cells arise simultaneously from the base of a whole field of columnar epithelium, not from single cells in an initial focus. **(b)** Two small fields of severe dysplastic squamous epithelium that are still covered by columnar cells. There is no active spread of the epithelium beyond the borders of the fields (hematoxylin and eosin).

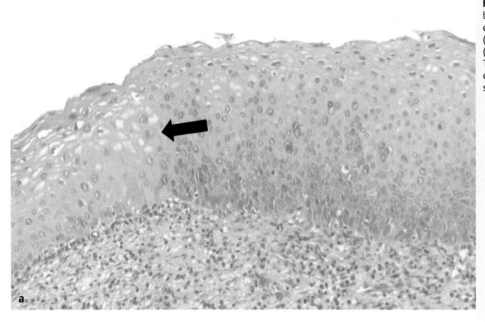

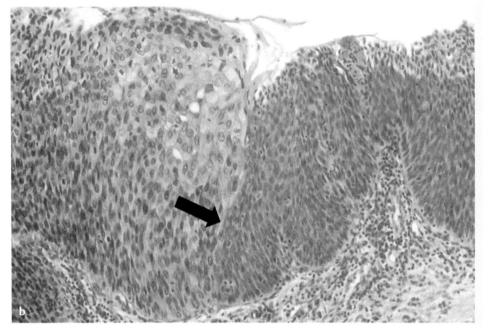

Fig. 1.10 (a–c) Different fields of SIL separated by sharp borders. (a) Border between squamous epithelium with permissive (productive) HPV infection (left) and slightly dysplastic squamous epithelium (LSIL) (right). (b) Border between two fields of HSIL. The borders are indicated by arrows (hematoxylin and eosin). (c) HSIL next to a typical condyloma with tall stromal papillae and marked koilocytosis.

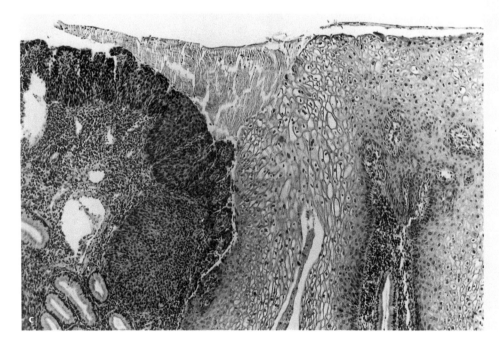

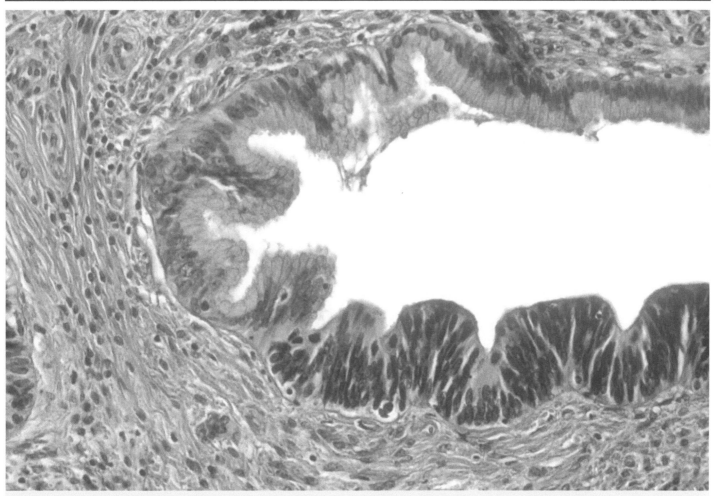

Fig. 1.11 Adenocarcinoma in situ. As in SIL, the border between atypical and normal columnar epithelium is abrupt (hematoxylin and eosin).

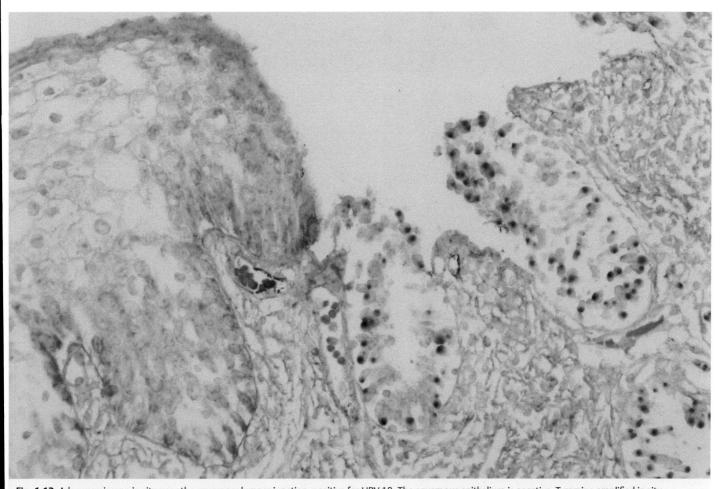

Fig. 1.12 Adenocarcinoma in situ near the squamocolumnar junction, positive for HPV 18. The squamous epithelium is negative. Tyramine amplified in situ hybridization. (This image is provided courtesy of S. Syrjänen.)

Further Reading

Ali H, Donovan B, Wand H, et al. Genital warts in young Australians five years into national human papillomavirus vaccination programme: national surveillance data. BMJ 2013;346:f2032

Dürst M, Gissmann L, Ikenberg H, zur Hausen H. A papillomavirus DNA from a cervical carcinoma and its prevalence in cancer biopsy samples from different geographic regions. Proc Natl Acad Sci U S A 1983;80:3812–3815

FUTURE II Study Group. Quadrivalent vaccine against human papillomavirus to prevent high-grade cervical lesions. N Engl J Med 2007;356:1915–1927

Garland SM, Hernandez-Avila M, Wheeler CM, et al. Females United to Unilaterally Reduce Endo/Ectocervical Disease (FUTURE) I Investigators. Quadrivalent vaccine against human papillomavirus to prevent anogenital diseases. N Engl J Med 2007;356: 1928–1943

Joura EA, Garland SM, Paavonen J, et al. FUTURE I and II Study Group. Effect of the human papillomavirus (HPV) quadrivalent vaccine in a subgroup of women with cervical and vulvar disease: retrospective pooled analysis of trial data. BMJ 2012;344:e1401

Joura EA, Giuliano AR, Iversen OE, et al. Broad Spectrum HPV Vaccine Study. A 9-valent HPV vaccine against infection and intraepithelial neoplasia in women. N Engl J Med 2015;372(8):711–723

Lehtinen M, Paavonen J, Wheeler CM, et al. HPV PATRICIA Study Group. Overall efficacy of HPV-16/18 AS04-adjuvanted vaccine against grade 3 or greater cervical intraepithelial neoplasia: 4-year end-of-study analysis of the randomised, double-blind PATRICIA trial. Lancet Oncol 2012;13:89–99

Paavonen J, Naud P, Salmerón J, et al. HPV PATRICIA Study Group. Efficacy of human papillomavirus (HPV)-16/18 AS04-adjuvanted vaccine against cervical infection and precancer caused by oncogenic HPV types (PATRICIA): final analysis of a double-blind, randomised study in young women. Lancet 2009;374:301–314

Reich O, Regauer S. Thin HSIL of the cervix: detecting a variant of high-grade squamous intraepithelial lesions with a p16INK4a antibody. Int J Gynecol Pathol 2016 (in press)

Ronco G, Dillner J, Elfström KM, et al. International HPV screening working group. Efficacy of HPV-based screening for prevention of invasive cervical cancer: follow-up of four European randomised controlled trials. Lancet 2014;383(9916):524–532

Schiffman M, Castle PE, Jeronimo J, Rodriguez AC, Wacholder S. Human papillomavirus and cervical cancer. Lancet 2007;370:890–907

Schiffman M, Solomon D. Clinical practice. Cervical-cancer screening with human papillomavirus and cytologic cotesting. N Engl J Med 2013;369:2324–2331

zur Hausen H. Condylomata acuminata and human genital cancer. Cancer Res 1976;36 (2, pt 2):794

Chapter 2

Role of Colposcopy

2 Role of Colposcopy

Colposcopy is a diagnostic procedure to visualize the epithelia of the lower genital tract with magnification and adequate illumination. Applications of acetic acid and Lugol's iodine (Schiller's test) are useful parts of the examination. The aim of colposcopy is to identify and plan the treatment of premalignant (intraepithelial) diseases of the cervix, vagina, vulva, and perianal region. Worldwide, colposcopy is performed in different settings and for different indications. Competency in colposcopy avoids overtreatment and promises better patient outcomes. Colposcopy can be applied in a variety of contexts.

2.1 Routine Colposcopy

We believe colposcopic inspection of the cervix should be an integral part of the gynecologic examination. This approach gives the examiner an appreciation of the dynamic processes that occur at the cervix at the different stages of life as well as experience and confidence in assessing colposcopic findings. All lesions—whether inflammatory, condylomas, polyps, preinvasive, or invasive—are better seen when magnified and optimally illuminated. With practice, the colposcopist can react quickly and accurately detect visible lesions. Many believe colposcopy should not be used as a screening method where the likelihood of finding cancer precursors is low, but it is easy to combine colposcopy with routine cytology. The diagnostic accuracy of cytology and colposcopy can then be assessed by performing a biopsy of colposcopically suspect findings. We believe this practice is superior to colposcopy restricted to evaluating abnormal smears because it can detect lesions missed by cytology. In contrast to cytology, colposcopy can localize suspicious lesions. If cytology is positive but the ectocervix and the vagina are normal, an endocervical lesion can be predicted. In this way, cytology can select patients for biopsy. Also, it is possible to direct a smear for cytology under colposcopic guidance so that a colposcopic lesion can be scraped directly with an Ayre's spatula, or the endocervical canal can be sampled when there are no lesions on the ectocervix. There is also no doubt that the quality of cytology can be improved by the simultaneous use of colposcopy. It is instructive to follow up on given patient over years.

2.2 Colposcopy to Evaluate an Abnormal Pap Smear

In many countries, colposcopy is used primarily to evaluate women with an abnormal Pap smear. Most countries use the Bethesda nomenclature for cervical cytology (Table 2.1). In this setting, the goal is to identify and localize lesions suspected on the basis of abnormal cytologic findings. In a meta-analysis, the sensitivity of colposcopy for the detection of high-grade squamous intraepithelial lesion (HSIL) was 96%, with a specificity of 48%. Table 2.2 shows the 2014 WHO histologic terminology for epithelial cervical neoplasia.

Colposcopy is no substitute for histologic evaluation, and a biopsy should be taken from the area of the most clinically severe abnormality of any lesion.

2.3 Colposcopy to Evaluate Patients Positive for HPV

Testing for high-risk types of human papillomavirus (HPV) is more sensitive for the detection of HSIL than cytology. The association between infection with high-risk types of HPV and HSIL and cervical cancer is so strong that HPV testing has become an important part of the management of women with cytologic abnormalities. Furthermore, the detection of HPV after treatment for HSIL is an accurate predictor of relapse, significantly more sensitive than repeated cytology.

The limitation of HPV testing is that women who test positive for high-risk (HR) HPV carry only a small risk of underlying HSIL or cancer. Dual staining for p16^{INK4a}/Ki-67 increases specificity and maintained sensitivity for the diagnosis of HSIL or adenocarcinoma in situ (AIS) compared with testing for HR-HPV. Most experts agree that women positive for both high-risk HPV and p16^{INK4a}/Ki-67 should be referred for colposcopy to verify or rule out a lesion.

Because there is a strong evidence base that HPV testing is advantageous in primary screening of women aged 30 years or older, HPV screening is coming to augment or supplant cytologic screening. This trend looks likely to spread worldwide so that we will likely see a large number of women positive for high-risk HPV referred for colposcopic evaluation of the cervix.

In women with low-grade cytologic smears, normal colposcopic findings are associated with a high negative predictive value, even in the presence of HPV infection.

2.4 Colposcopy to Evaluate Abnormal Cytologic Findings during Pregnancy

Colposcopy is safe in pregnancy and is performed with the intention of ruling out invasive cancer. Cumulative data suggest that expectant treatment of pregnant women with an abnormal Pap smear (i.e., delaying treatment of preinvasive changes until after pregnancy) is safe.

2.5 Colposcopy to Evaluate Lesions before Treatment

Colposcopy is performed before treatment of presumed intraepithelial lesions to exclude overt invasive cancer and define the extent of disease. Also, colposcopy is helpful to plan the extent of conization and reduce the risk of overly aggressive excisions in young patients.

2.6 Colposcopy in Screen-and-Treat Approaches in Resource-Poor Settings

In developing countries with high rates of mortality from cervical cancer, new algorithms for cervical screening are being tested. These algorithms include high-risk HPV testing with consecutive colposcopy of HPV-positive women and immediate treatment if a lesion is detected.

Table 2.1 The 2014 Bethesda System for reporting cervical cytology

Specimen Type

Indicate conventional smear (Pap smear) vs. liquid based preparation vs. other

Specimen Adequacy

• Satisfactory for evaluation *(describe presence or absence of endocervical/transformation zone component and any other quality indicators, e.g., partially obscuring blood, inflammation, etc.)*

• Unsatisfactory for evaluation… *(specify reason)*

 – Specimen rejected/not processed *(specify reason)*

 – Specimen processed and examined, but unsatisfactory for evaluation of epithelial abnormality because of *(specify reason)*

General Categorization (optional)

• Negative for intraepithelial lesion or malignancy

• Other: see Interpretation/Results *(e.g. endometrial cells in a woman ≥45 years of age)*

• Epithelial Cell Abnormality: See Interpretation/Results *(specify* 'squamous' *or* 'glandular' *as appropriate)*

Interpretation/Result

Negative for Intraepithelial Lesion or Malignancy

(When there is no cellular evidence of neoplasia, state this in the General Categorization above and/or in the Interpretation/Result section of the report–whether or not there are organisms or other non-neoplastic findings)

Non-Neoplastic Findings *(optional to report; list not inclusive)*

• Non-neoplastic cellular variations

 – Squamous metaplasia

 – Keratotic changes

 – Tubal metaplasia

 – Atrophy

 – Pregnancy-associated changes

• Reactive cellular changes associated with:

 – Inflammation (includes typical repair)

 ▪ Lymphocytic (follicular) cervicitis

 – Radiation

 – Intrauterine contraceptive device (IUD)

• Glandular cells status post – hysterectomy

Organisms

• *Trichomonas vaginalis*

• Fungal organisms morphologically consistent with *Candida* spp.

• Shift in flora suggestive for bacterial vaginosis

• Bacteria morphologically consistent with *Actinomyces* spp.

• Cellular changes consistent with herpes simplex virus

• Cellular changes consistent with cytomegalovirus

Other

• Endometrial cells *(in a woman ≥45 years of age)*
 (Specify if negative for squamous intraepithelial lesion)

Epithelial Cell Abnormalities

Squamous Cell

• Atypical squamous cells

 – of undetermined significance (ASC-US)

 – cannot exclude HSIL (ASC-H)

• Low-grade squamous intraepithelial lesion (LSIL)
 (encompassing: HPV/mild dysplasia/CIN1)

• High-grade squamous intraepithelial lesion (HSIL)
 (encompassing: moderate and severe dysplasia, CIS; CIN2 and CIN3)

 – with features suspicious for invasion (if invasion is suspected)

• Squamous cell carcinoma

(continued)

Table 2.1 The 2014 Bethesda System for Reporting Cervical Cytology *(continued)*

Glandular Cell

- Atypical
  - Endocervical cells *(NOS or specify in comments)*
  - Endometrial cells *(NOS or specify in comments)*
  - Glandular cells *(NOS or specify in comments)*
- Atypical
  - Endocervical cells, favor neoplastic
  - Glandular cells, favor neoplastic
- Endocervical adenocarcinoma in situ
- Adenocarcinoma
  - Endocervical
  - Endometrial
  - Extrauterine
  - Not otherwise specified (NOS)

Other malignant neoplasms: (specify)

Adjunctive Testing

Provide a brief description of the test method(s) and report the results so that it is easily understood by the clinician

Computer-assisted interpretation of clinical cytology

If case examined by an automated device, specify devise and result

Educational notes and comments appended to cytology reports *(optional)*

Suggestions should be concise and consistent with clinical follow-up guidelines published by professional organizations (references to relevant publications may be included)

Abbreviation: CIN, cervical intraepithelial neoplasia; CIS, carcinoma in situ; HPV, human papillomavirus; NOS, not otherwise specified; Pap, Papanicolaou.

Table 2.2 Terminologies for squamous and glandular cervical precursor lesions

Older classification	WHO classification (2003)	WHO classification (2014)
Mild dysplasia	CIN 1	Low-grade squamous intraepithelial lesion (LSIL)
Moderate dysplasia Severe dysplasia/carcinoma in situ	CIN 2 CIN 3	High-grade squamous intraepithelial lesion (HSIL)
Endocervical glandular dysplasia	Adenocarcinoma in situ (AIS)	Adenocarcinoma in situ (AIS) (syn: high-grade cervical glandular intraepithelial neoplasia [HG-CIGN])

Further Reading

Bosgraaf RP, Mast PP, Struik-van der Zanden PH, Bulten J, Massuger LF, Bekkers RL. Overtreatment in a see-and-treat approach to cervical intraepithelial lesions. Obstet Gynecol 2013;121(6):1209–1216

Cantor SB, Cárdenas-Turanzas M, Cox DD, et al. Accuracy of colposcopy in the diagnostic setting compared with the screening setting. Obstet Gynecol 2008;111:7–14

Deodhar K, Sankaranarayanan R, Jayant K, et al. Accuracy of concurrent visual and cytology screening in detecting cervical cancer precursors in rural India. Int J Cancer 2012;131(6):E954–E962

Gage JC, Hanson VW, Abbey K, et al; ASCUS LSIL Triage Study (ALTS) Group. Number of cervical biopsies and sensitivity of colposcopy. Obstet Gynecol 2006;108(2):264–272

International Federation of Cervical Pathology and Colposcopy. www.ifcpc.org/en/education

Kelly RS, Walker P, Kitchener H, Moss SM. Incidence of cervical intraepithelial neoplasia grade 2 or worse in colposcopy-negative/human papillomavirus-positive women with low-grade cytological abnormalities. BJOG 2012;119:20–25

Kurman RJ, Carcangiu ML, Herrington S, Young RH. WHO Classification of Tumours of Female Reproductive Organs. Lyon: IARC press; 2014

Kyrgiou M, Tsoumpou I, Vrekoussis T, et al. The up-to-date evidence on colposcopy practice and treatment of cervical intraepithelial neoplasia: the Cochrane colposcopy & cervical cytopathology collaborative group (C5 group) approach. Cancer Treat Rev 2006;32(7):516–523

Leeson SC, Alibegashvili T, Arbyn M, et al. The future role for colposcopy in Europe. J Low Genit Tract Dis 2014;18(1):70–78

Mitchell MF, Schottenfeld D, Tortolero-Luna G, Cantor SB, Richards-Kortum R. Colposcopy for the diagnosis of squamous intraepithelial lesions: a meta-analysis. Obstet Gynecol 1998;91(4):626–631

Nayar R, Wilbur DC. The Bethesda System for Reporting Cervical Cytology. Cham: Springer; 2015

Petry KU, Schmidt D, Scherbring S, et al. Triaging Pap cytology negative, HPV positive cervical cancer screening results with p16/Ki-67 Dual-stained cytology. Gynecol Oncol 2011;121(3):505–509

Tatti S, Bornstein J, Prendiville W. Colposcopy: a global perspective: introduction of the new IFCPC colposcopy terminology. Obstet Gynecol Clin North Am 2013;40(2):235–250

Underwood M, Arbyn M, Parry-Smith W, et al. Accuracy of colposcopy-directed punch biopsies: a systematic review and meta-analysis. BJOG 2012;119(11):1293–1301

Chapter 3

The Colposcope and the Colposcopic Examination

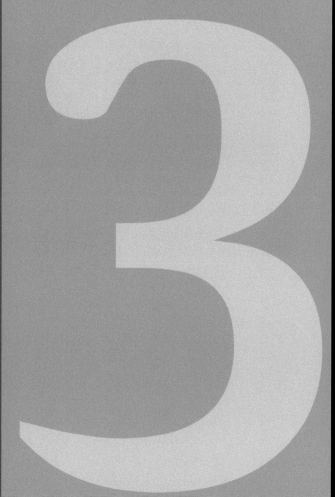

3 The Colposcope and the Colposcopic Examination

Modern colposcopes permit magnification between ×6 and ×40. Magnification ×10 is most suitable for routine use. Higher magnifications reveal minor features but are not necessary for accurate diagnosis. The colposcope can be equipped with a green filter to filter out red and thereby enhance the vascular appearance of the vessels by making them look darker.

A colposcope can be mounted in different ways. For routine use, a swivel arm attached to the gynecologic examination chair is very practical (Fig. 3.1). The scope can be easily adjusted by hand, both vertically and horizontally. A colposcope on a mobile stand is independent of the examination table (Fig. 3.2). It can be fitted with a swivel arm and, with the wheels locked, can be used in the same way as a scope mounted on the examination table. Colposcopes mounted on the wall or ceiling are easy to handle because of their mobility. The head of the colposcope can be tilted up, down, and sideways. There is usually no need for the fine adjustment, as a sharp focus can be achieved just as easily by positioning the scope at the working distance of 20 to 24 cm.

Photographic and video equipment are important accessories. For teaching, a camera and video equipment are mandatory. Video colposcopy can improve patient satisfaction. New technologies are likely to improve the colposcopic detection of precancerous lesions.

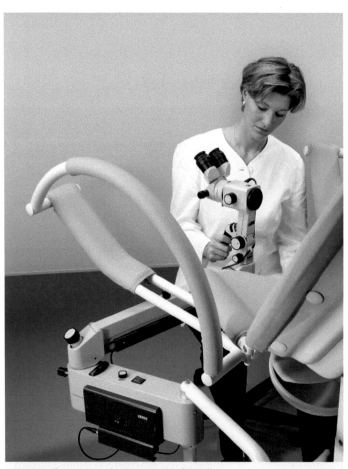

Fig. 3.1 Chair-mounted colposcope (Carl Zeiss).

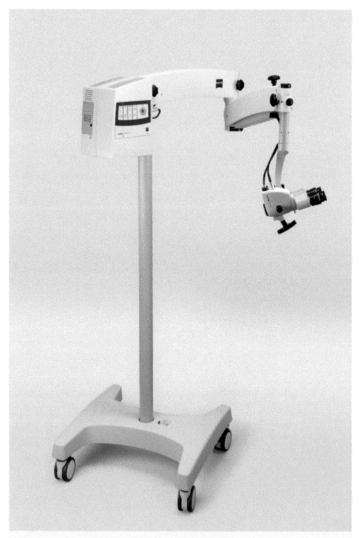

Fig. 3.2 Colposcope mounted on a stand (Carl Zeiss).

3.1 Colposcopic Instruments

Colposcopy requires few instruments. In addition to the colposcope, one needs a duckbill speculum or Breisky-type retractors, anatomic forceps and swabs, dilute acetic acid and iodine, and biopsy instruments (Fig. 3.3). Some colposcopists use an endocervical speculum to improve access to the cervical canal (Fig. 3.3).

3.1.1 Specula

A duckbill speculum (Fig. 3.3) usually provides adequate exposure of the cervix and can be manipulated by the examiner without assistance. Duckbill specula are available in various sizes. On occasion, vaginal (Breisky) retractors (Fig. 3.3) are helpful, particularly to evaluate lesions involving the fornix and vagina. A disadvantage of the Breisky speculum is that the anterior blade needs to be held by an assistant.

3.1.2 Forceps

Anatomic forceps 20 cm or longer are needed to handle swabs (Fig. 3.3). They are more practical than tenacula. Sometimes forceps can be used to improve access to the cervical canal, for example, to evaluate the squamocolumnar junction (SCJ) and define the type of transformation zone.

3.1.3 Containers

Swabs are placed in a bowl from which they can be easily retrieved with forceps. For the acetic acid test (Fig. 3.3), swabs are soaked in 3% acetic acid and handled with forceps. Iodine (Lugol's solution) is put into test tubes, which are placed in a rack. Tampons, which can be removed by the patient later (Fig. 3.12), are available.

3.2 Biopsy Instruments

There are several types of biopsy instruments (Fig. 3.3). They are usually scissor-shaped and between 20 and 25 cm in length.

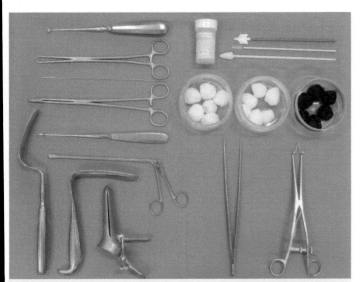

Fig. 3.3 Instruments for colposcopy (clockwise from lower left): Breisky specula, biopsy forceps, curet, oval forceps, Chrobak's probe, tenacula, sharp curet, ThinPrep container, three cytobrushes, swabs for acetic acid and iodine, cervical dilator according to Cogan, and anatomic forceps.

Sharp curets of various sizes are needed for scraping the endocervical canal and to obtain material from clinically invasive cancers. To curet a narrow endocervical canal, instruments with fine, sharp grooves are more practical than spoon-shaped ones.

3.2.1 Tenacula

To prevent slipping of the biopsy punch and obtain an accurately directed biopsy, fixation of the cervix is sometimes helpful. This can be done easily and painlessly with a single-toothed tenaculum (Fig. 3.3). Cervical polyps can be avulsed with polyp forceps (Fig. 3.3).

3.2.2 Chrobak's Probe

Chrobak's probe (Fig. 3.4) is a thin steel sound with a bulbous head that is useful to distinguish between carcinomas and papillomas or flat ectocervical ulcers. When investigating normal tissue or benign tumors, the probe encounters an elastic resistance; in contrast, malignant tissue feels soft, like warm butter.

3.3 The Colposcopic Examination

The colposcopic examination begins with an explanation for the patient. Video systems make this easier. The vulva and perianal region are inspected. An appropriate duckbill speculum is inserted; lubrication of the speculum can be helpful. Secretions and signs of inflammation in the vagina are noted, if present. The cervix is visualized and dry swabbed to remove mucous. The cervix, particularly the vessels, is inspected colposcopically in the native state. A smear for cervical cytology (Pap smear) is obtained with an Ayre's spatula, cervical brush, or cotton-tipped swab. If indicated, material for human papillomavirus (HPV) testing is obtained with an appropriate brush. If liquid-based cytology is used, only one sample of material is obtained with an appropriate brush and transferred to the container; cytology, HPV testing, and other molecular tests are done from the liquid suspension.

On occasion, the cervix can be difficult to expose adequately. This can be the case in very obese women, patients with a narrow vagina or vaginal stenosis, or patients with pelvic tumors or a fibroid uterus distorting the anatomy. In these (rare) cases, we obtain a smear without visualizing the cervix proper.

The acetic acid test and the iodine test (Schiller's test), which we consider integral parts of the colposcopic examination, are next. At the end of the colposcopic examination, we make a decision as to whether and where to biopsy. It is our practice to biopsy a major lesion noted at colposcopy without awaiting the results of cytology or HPV testing.

3.3.1 Application of Acetic Acid

Application of 3% acetic acid plays a decisive role in colposcopic diagnostics. No colposcopic examination is complete without it.

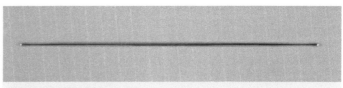

Fig. 3.4 Chrobak's probe.

After removing vaginal secretions with dry swabs, the cervical epithelium is often still masked by a film of mucus, especially in the presence of ectopy. Cleansing the cervix of mucous with acetic acid enhances the colposcopic features. This applies especially to the grapelike structure of columnar epithelium in ectopy. However, all epithelial lesions become more distinct with acetic acid, the color changes are accentuated, and the various structures become more easily distinguishable from one another (Fig. 3.5). Care should be taken to apply the swab with acetic acid for 10 seconds or longer; if there is any question, application of acetic acid should be repeated.

Ectopy shows a dramatic change of color after application of acetic acid. The intense dark red ectopic columnar epithelium becomes paler and displays shades of pink to white. At the same time, the grapelike structures become more pronounced because of swelling and enlargement of the villi (Fig. 3.6).

Similar changes can be seen in altered epithelia. The epithelial swelling caused by acetic acid turns atypical epithelium white and accentuates its surface contour (Fig. 3.7). The patterns of mosaic and punctation also become more distinct, and the red partitions and fine petechiae stand out against the white epithelium (Fig. 3.8).

Because the effect on pathologic epithelium is not as rapid as on ectopic columnar epithelium, the white epithelium that appears after application of acetic acid should not be confused with leukoplakia.

3.3.2 Schiller's (Iodine) Test

Application of iodine quickly produces intense staining of glycogen-containing epithelium (Fig. 3.1). This makes it an important

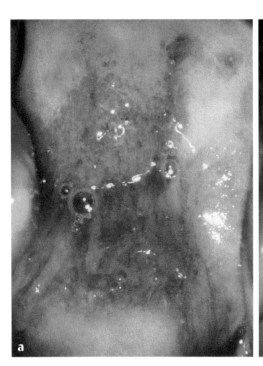
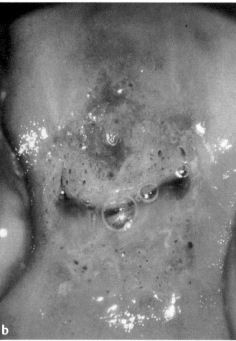

Fig. 3.5 (a) Normal transformation zone before application of acetic acid. The fine details are clouded by mucous. **(b)** Removal of the mucous with 3% acetic acid reveals numerous gland openings.

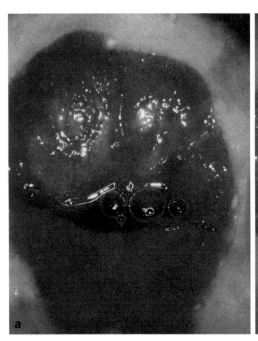
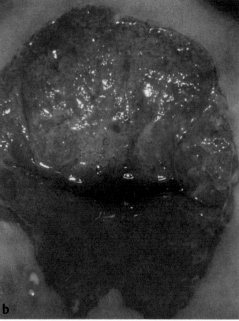

Fig. 3.6 (a) Large intensely red area around external os. The border to the normal squamous epithelium is abrupt. **(b)** Application of 3% acetic acid evokes the grapelike structure of the mucosa covered by columnar epithelium. Note the blanching of the previously intensely red area caused by the swelling of the columnar epithelium. Individual gland openings in the adjacent squamous epithelium on the posterior lip indicate that transformation has occurred.

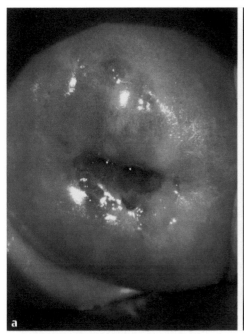 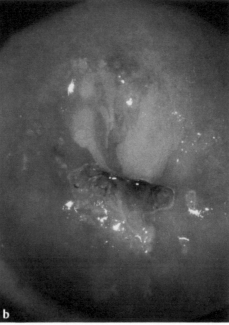

Fig. 3.7 (a) A distinct red area on the anterior lip of the external os. On the posterior lip, there is a small intensely red area. **(b)** Application of 3% acetic acid reveals several sharply demarcated white areas on the anterior lip. There are some cuffed gland openings near the white areas. Histology showed HSIL (CIN 2). The area on the posterior lip is columnar epithelium with a narrow transformation zone at its edge.

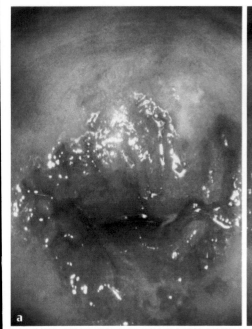 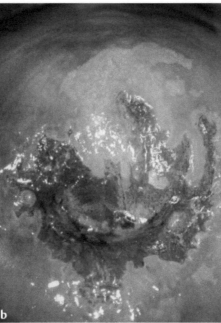

Fig. 3.8 (a) Before application of acetic acid, the transformation zone is inconspicuous. The experienced colposcopist will detect an early lesion at 12 o'clock position outside the transformation zone. **(b)** The white color and mosaic pattern of HSIL (CIN 3) are due to cellular edema caused by acetic acid.

diagnostic aid for assessing colposcopic findings. Lugol's iodine solution was first used in clinical diagnosis by Walter Schiller in 1929, hence the term Schiller's test. While some colposcopists do not use iodine, we find it very useful for the evaluation of colposcopic morphology. We pay particular attention to how aceto-white epithelium reacts with the Lugol's solution (Table 3.1).

The 1% iodine solution consists of 2 g iodine and 4 g potassium iodide dissolved in 200 mL distilled water.

The Schiller's test depends on the interaction between iodine and glycogen. The glycogen-containing vaginal epithelium of women of reproductive age quickly takes up iodine to produce an intense mahogany brown. Glycogen-free epithelium stains yellow (not brown) with iodine (Fig. 3.9). Such an area is referred to as iodine-yellow (sometimes—and in our opinion incorrectly—to as iodine negative).

Iodine solution stains normal glycogen-containing squamous epithelium uniformly deep brown. Such epithelium is found during the reproductive period and reflects the influence of estrogens (Fig. 3.10).

Columnar epithelium does not stain with iodine (Fig. 3.10) nor does thin regenerating epithelium, seen during the early stages of squamous metaplasia (Fig. 3.11). Failure to stain with iodine is useful to assess inflammatory lesions, which, because of their increased vascularity and capillary dilatation, can mimic punctation. Inflammation is associated with indistinct margins and failure to react strongly with iodine (Fig. 3.12).

Dysplastic epithelium stains with iodine as described later, even when still thin. This is an important difference between the normal transformation zone and the acetowhite epithelium. A colposcopic lesion, as well as the whole length of the vagina, can display all shades between tan and the chestnut brown of normal squamous epithelium (Fig. 3.13).

The vagina can have a stippled brown appearance, especially after menopause, when the effect of estrogen wanes. The

Table 3.1 Normal and abnormal reactions with iodine

Designation	Staining	Underlying histology
Iodine positive	Deep brown (mahogany)	Mature glycogen-containing squamous epithelium
Iodine negative	None	Columnar epithelium Immature metaplastic epithelium Inflammation
Weak staining	Lighter shades of brown	Waning estrogen effect (menopause) Transformation zone during metaplasia
Iodine-yellow	Characteristic canary yellow to ocher	HSIL (CIN 2, CIN 3)
Nonsuspicious iodine-yellow area	Yellow	Metaplastic squamous epithelium LSIL (CIN 1)
Iodine positive mosaic or punctation	Brown, brownish, speckled brown	Condylomatous colpitis, condylomatous lesions

Abbreviations: CIN, cervical intraepithelial neoplasia; HSIL, high-grade squamous intraepithelial lesion; LSIL, low-grade squamous intraepithelial lesion.

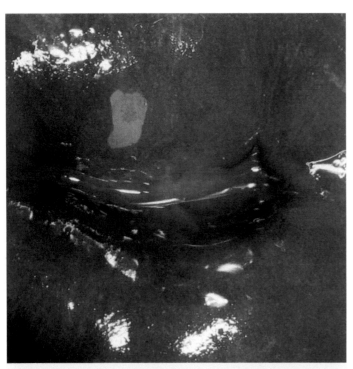

Fig. 3.9 Original squamous epithelium displays uniform mahogany staining with iodine. Note a sharply demarcated iodine-yellow area at the 11 o'clock position.

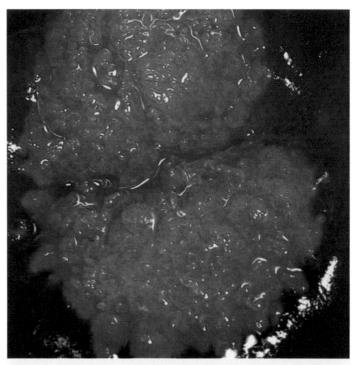

Fig. 3.10 The columnar epithelium of an ectopy does not stain with iodine (iodine negative). It shows only a slight discoloration due to the thin film of solution veiling it. The original epithelium stains characteristically deep brown.

postmenopausal cervix and vagina stain light brown to yellow (Fig. 3.14; see also Fig. 6.7).

The various shades of brown of the normal transformation zone depend on the maturity (i.e., the glycogen content) of the squamous epithelium (Fig. 3.15). The squamous epithelium in the fully developed transformation zone stains mahogany brown. The transformation zone in such cases can be recognized only by the gland openings and the retention cysts (Fig. 3.16). The deep brown color distinguishes it from the acetowhite epithelium, as metaplastic and dysplastic epithelia are almost always glycogen-free.

Iodine solution typically reacts with squamous intraepithelial lesion (SIL) to produce a characteristic ocher yellow (Figs. 3.16–3.20). In some cases, only portions of the transformation zone stain yellow (Fig. 3.20). Such areas should be regarded with suspicion, should be carefully searched for, and should be considered for biopsy.

The colposcopist who uses the Schiller's test routinely will often see well-demarcated areas with a characteristic canary yellow color that otherwise escape colposcopic detection. Such an area, which is otherwise inconspicuous, is referred to as a nonsuspicious iodine-yellow area, and is usually due to metaplastic squamous epithelium (Fig. 3.9). If the exact location of a nonsuspicious iodine-yellow area has been noted, colposcopic examination after the effect of iodine has subsided can detect a subtle color difference between this area and normal squamous epithelium (Fig. 6.84).

Not only the nuances of color, but also the borders between normal and altered epithelia can be viewed to advantage with the help of iodine. The epithelial borders within colposcopic lesions also become distinct (Fig. 3.8; see also Fig. 6.142). There is no better way to demonstrate the sharpness and clarity of epithelial borders. This is of great diagnostic import, as poorly circumscribed colposcopic areas are hardly ever significant (Figs. 3.10–3.13 and 3.15).

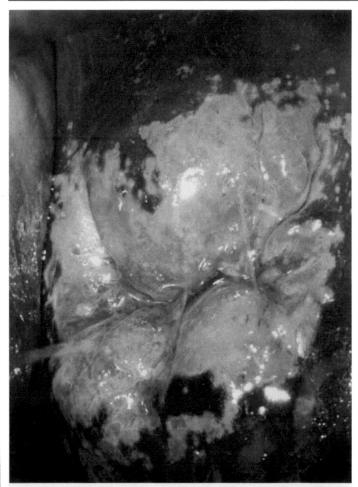

Fig. 3.11 The normal transformation zone does not stain with iodine. Note the contrast with the mahogany color of the original squamous epithelium.

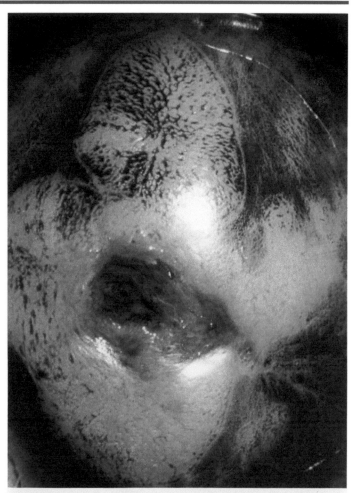

Fig. 3.13 This transformation zone has a stippled appearance with iodine reflecting the various stages of development of the metaplastic epithelium.

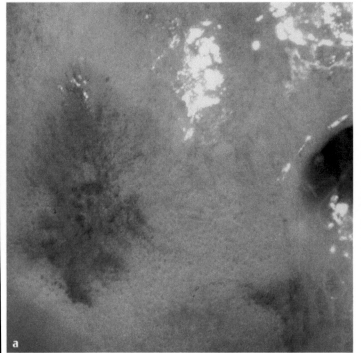

a

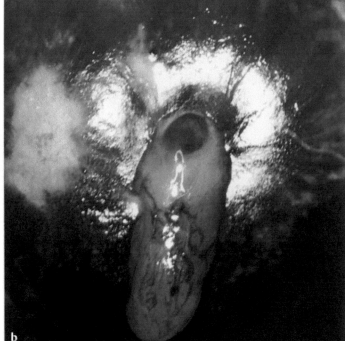

b

Fig. 3.12 (a) Red, inflamed area lateral to the external os. (b) This area does not stain with iodine and is poorly demarcated from the adjacent deep brown original epithelium.

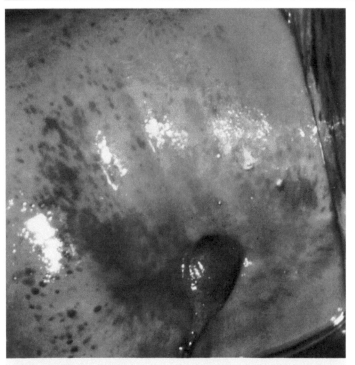

Fig. 3.14 Yellowish light brown of atrophic epithelium after application of iodine. At least some of the dark spots are due to subepithelial hemorrhages.

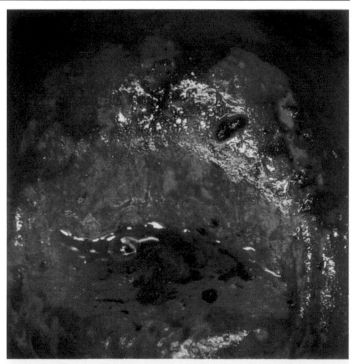

Fig. 3.15 When transformation is more advanced, various shades of brown may appear, according to the maturity of the metaplastic epithelium.

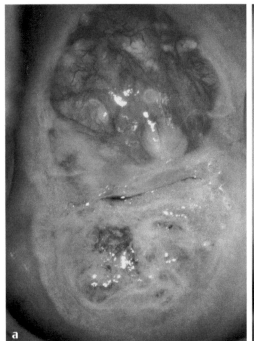

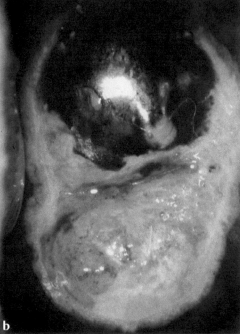

Fig. 3.16 (a) Very different appearance of the transformation zones anteriorly and posteriorly. On the anterior lip, the squamous epithelium is attenuated over retention (nabothian) cysts, and blood vessels coarse over their surfaces. The posterior lip shows acetowhite epithelium and gland openings. **(b)** Surprising reaction with iodine. The epithelium covering the retention cysts is fully mature and contains glycogen. The area on the posterior lip, which stains partly or not at all with iodine, corresponded to HSIL (CIN 3) histologically.

3.4 Therapeutic Implications of Abnormal Colposcopic Findings

Abnormal or suspicious colposcopic findings should be evaluated by biopsy under direct colposcopic guidance. It is important that treatment is based on a histologic diagnosis, not on a colposcopic finding or a cytologic result. Cytology shows only whether epithelial atypia is present, and cytology imprecisely predicts histology. HPV testing is a useful adjunct.

3.4.1 Benign Colposcopic Findings

Ectopy

Ectopy is columnar mucosa on the ectocervix. The border between the columnar epithelium and the squamous epithelium of the cervix is called the squamocolumnar junction (SCJ). A large ectopy can produce symptoms, such as mucous discharge and postcoital contact bleeding. Symptomatic ectopy can be treated, particularly in women who have completed their

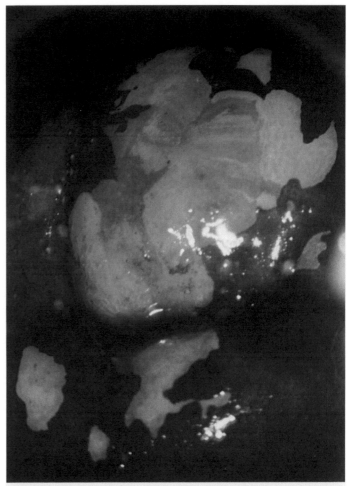

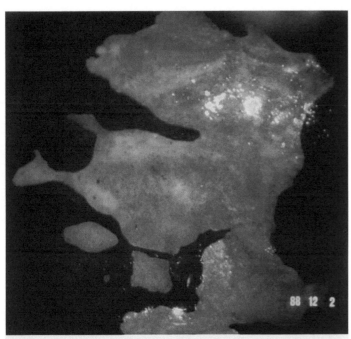

Fig. 3.17 Nonsuspicious iodine-yellow area. The lesion is sharply demarcated and in the same plane as its surroundings. Histology showed metaplastic squamous epithelium.

Fig. 3.18 Nonsuspicious iodine-yellow area with different color tones, from yellow to brown, corresponding to sharply demarcated epithelial fields. Histology showed metaplastic squamous epithelium.

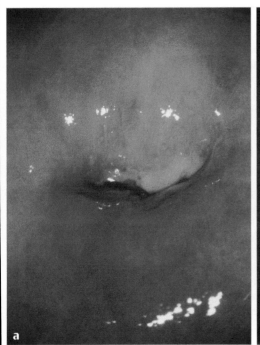

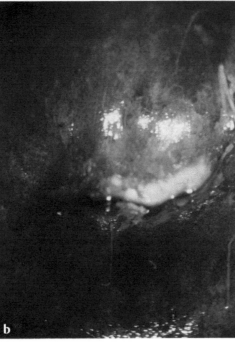

Fig. 3.19 (a) Application of 3% acetic acid reveals a small, easily missed white area on the anterior external os. **(b)** After application of iodine, the area on the external os appears bright yellow. Histology showed HSIL (CIN 2) in the cervical canal.

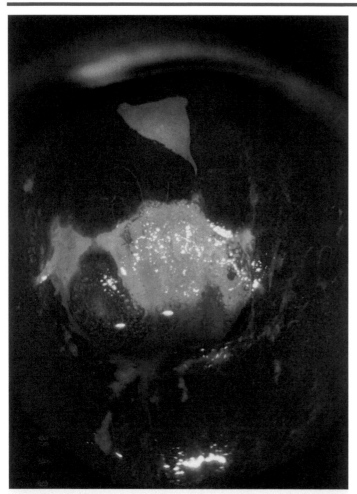

Fig. 3.20 Patchy uptake of iodine by a partially atypical transformation zone. Histology showed HSIL (CIN 3). On the left, within the transformation zone, there is a small condylomatous area with iodine-positive punctation. At 12 o'clock position, there is an isolated nonsuspicious iodine-yellow area.

Condylomatous Lesions

Several medical and ablative options are available to treat condylomas. We prefer laser ablation. With a laser, lesions of the cervix, vagina, and vulva can be vaporized under direct colposcopic guidance. Papillary and spiked condylomas can be surgically ablated. Papillary lesions, and extensive flat ones, can be removed with a diathermy loop with the current set low enough that the underlying tissue is not damaged. Flat condylomas near papillary lesions can also be removed with a diathermy loop or cauterized after biopsy. Diathermy of the base of the lesion is important to help prevent recurrences due to residual infected tissue.

Cryosurgery can also be used. Spiked condylomas adjacent to lesions treated with cryosurgery have been observed to regress spontaneously, presumably due to an immune response induced by the freezing.

In patients with flat condylomas, invasive carcinoma should be ruled out with biopsy. If the surface of the lesion is particularly coarse, then it can have an endophytic component, and the depth of treatment should be increased to help prevent recurrence. If the biopsy shows atypia, the lesion should be treated as intraepithelial neoplasia.

Medical options for the treatment of condylomas include imiquimod and podophyllotoxin. Because of the risk of recurrence, these substances are also used for the adjuvant treatment after surgical ablation. Interferon-α hydrogel or 5-fluorouracil is seldom used.

3.4.2 Treatment of Premalignant (Intraepithelial) Cervical Lesions

Low-grade squamous intraepithelial lesion (LSIL, CIN 1) can and should be managed with short-term follow-up because such lesions can regress, especially if poorly demarcated colposcopically. A well-defined lesion persisting for approximately 1 to 2 years should be treated as a high-grade lesion. The aim of treatment is to remove or destroy the atypical epithelium in its entirety. Definitive treatment should be based on a precise definition of the lesion.

The following are diagnostic considerations in SIL (CIN):
- Histologic appearance.
- Extent of superficial spread, including extension into the endocervical canal.
- Depth of involvement of cervical glands (crypts).
- Exclusion of invasion.

Recent studies have addressed medical treatment for CIN (SIL).

Diagnostic Prerequisites

None of the first-line diagnostic methods (cytology, colposcopy, even guided biopsy) can be relied on absolutely for an accurate diagnosis of SIL (Table 3.2). Colposcopy can evaluate only the extent of the lesion on the surface, and only when the lesions are limited to the ectocervix. The endocervical speculum can visualize the lower portion of the canal, but lesions higher in the canal are out of reach of the colposcope. The colposcopic criteria for evaluating epithelia are not sufficiently accurate for decisions regarding treatment. Also, microinvasive carcinomas can be diagnosed colposcopically only when they have reached a certain size and are located on the ectocervix and not too far under the surface.

The diagnostic accuracy of colposcopically guided biopsies depends entirely on the sites from which they are taken, which in turn is determined by the colposcopic impression. Biopsy cannot always detect glandular involvement or invasion. Endocervical curettage shows only extension of SIL (CIN) into the cervical

families. In young women in whom ectopy is unusually large due to oral contraceptives, an alternate form of contraception can be considered. Ectopy can be ablated or removed with shallow excision, diathermy, cryosurgery, or laser treatment. With any method, the end result should be re-epithelialization with normal glycogen-containing squamous epithelium. In favorable cases, the SCJ will lie at the external os. Before treatment, care must be taken to rule out SIL or invasive disease by using cytology, histology, or HPV testing.

Normal Transformation Zone

The transformation zone per se is a normal finding and does not require treatment.

Metaplastic Epithelium with Leukoplakia, Punctation, or Mosaic

Leukoplakia, punctation, and mosaic should be evaluated with HPV testing and cytology and occasionally biopsy. If the findings are normal, the patient can be reassured. These patients do not need treatment or more intensive follow-up. Colposcopic findings resulting from metaplastic epithelium tend to be stable, as long-term follow-up studies show little change in the contours or cytology.

Table 3.2 Morphologic methods for evaluating cervical intraepithelial neoplasia

	Cytology	Colposcopy	Guided biopsy	Endocervical curettage	Conization
Histology	+	–	+ +	+ +	+ + +
Surface extent	–	+	+	+	+ + +
Glandular involve-ment	–	+	+	+	+ + +
Exclusion of invasion	–	–	+	+	+ + +

canal. It is not always possible to establish or rule out invasion or to determine the extent of glandular involvement and the depth of the crypts in the fragmented specimens obtained using biopsy techniques.

A definitive diagnosis of a high-grade squamous intraepithelial lesion (HSIL) requires complete excision of the abnormal area by conization (diathermy loop or cold knife) and rigorous histologic examination. Some guidelines consider adolescents and young women a special population to be considered for conservative management of HSIL.

Ablative Treatment of Squamous Intraepithelial Neoplasia

Ablative modalities performed in the office are attractive for patients, physicians, and payers, but they have to be used with an appreciation of their limitations and an understanding of cervical pathology. Colposcopy was widely used in the ablative treatment of SIL (CIN) in the hope that the lesions could be accurately destroyed with electrocoagulation diathermy, cryosurgery, or laser ablation. The idea was to reduce the number of cold-knife conizations, many of which had been performed without proper indications. Certainly, total destruction of the abnormal epithelium should achieve cure. If this result could be guaranteed, any ablative modality could be used; but the crux of the matter is that it is not possible to be sure that all abnormal epithelium has truly been destroyed.

Only lesions that are predominantly ectocervical and for which the entire SCJ is visible are suitable for superficial ablative treatment. Lesions reaching farther up into the cervical canal cannot be reached with certainty. There is also a risk of persisting dysplastic epithelium in deep glands (Fig. 3.21). Finally, microinvasive carcinomas can arise from the base of crypts, with no connection to any atypical epithelium on the surface. Such invasive tumors can extend deeper than 5 mm into the stroma and can also arise in unexpected places (Fig. 3.22).

The likelihood of deep extension and invasion is related to the extension of the lesion on the surface. In general, only large lesions are invasive. Deep extension in glands is less likely with low-grade lesions than with HSIL because HSIL develops more often from squamous metaplasia within the gland field and its crypts. Glandular involvement is impossible in regions of the original squamous epithelium.

Ablative modalities should be used only if the following criteria are met:
- The lesion is limited to LSIL.
- The lesion is small.
- The surface of the lesion is smooth.
- The lesion is located purely on the ectocervix.

The entire SCJ is visible. It is a misconception that regular follow-up after conservative treatment of SIL will detect any persistent or recurrent abnormality eventually. SIL can persistent in glands, as can a deep microinvasive carcinoma with no con-

nection to the surface of the remodeled cervix. Neither cytology nor colposcopy is appropriate for these contingencies, and these lesions will become manifest only when invasive disease breaks through the surface of the cervix.

Recurrence after superficial ablative therapy and three negative follow-up examinations is rare, but residual, mostly preinvasive, disease after conservative treatment is not infrequent. For this reason, cryosurgery is no longer considered appropriate for treating HSIL. The recurrence rate is inversely proportional to the depth of destruction. The amount of tissue damage required is comparable to that obtained with adequate excision, but conservative methods destroy the tissue and eliminate the possibility of examining the histology.

Invasive carcinoma and death of disease after conservative treatment of SIL have been reported but are rare. In expert hands, the results of superficial ablative methods are excellent. Finally, ablative treatment modalities have lost ground to loop excisional procedures, which are also performed on an outpatient basis and provide a good specimen for pathology.

Excisional Modalities: Loop Excision and Conization

Conization, whether with diathermy or a scalpel, is frequently a therapeutic as well as a diagnostic procedure. Further treatment depends on the quality of the histologic examination and on whether the lesion has been removed completely. Poor techniques have led to unnecessary complications. Treatment of patients after conization depends on the nature of the lesion in the cone and on the status of the margins of the cone.

Complete Excision

If the lesion is purely intraepithelial or early invasive with virtually no metastatic potential, nothing further apart from careful follow-up needs be done. HPV testing is increasingly being used in the follow-up of patients after conization.

Incomplete Excision

Excision is incomplete if the margins pass through at least LSIL, but this does not necessarily mean that major lesions have remained in the residual cervix. Coagulation of the wound surface after excisional procedures probably ablates residual intraepithelial neoplasia, the margin of excision can pass very close to the edge of a lesion, and small portions of residual atypical epithelium can be sloughed during the healing process.

Further management depends on several factors:
- Which margins are not clear (endocervical, ectocervical, or lateral)?
- How far from the margins of the lesion are the invasive foci?
- HPV status at follow-up.
- Is preservation of the uterus desired?

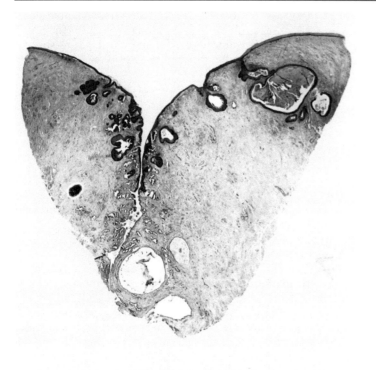

Fig. 3.21 Conization specimen. The surface of both lips of the cervix is covered by HSIL (CIN 3). Note the abrupt change at the junction with normal squamous epithelium. The HSIL involves glands and extends into the lower portion of the canal. On the right, there is extensive involvement of glands, which extend 10 mm under the surface. Such a lesion cannot be detected or suspected colposcopically.

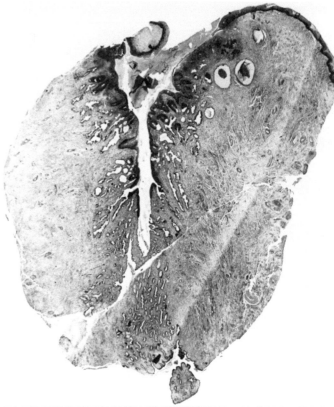

Fig. 3.22 Conization specimen. The right lip harbors a microinvasive carcinoma 2 mm in diameter. The surface and the glands show HSIL (CIN 3). The CIN on the left extends to the margin.

Cases in which the ectocervical margin is not clear are easiest to manage. In these patients, a persistent abnormality can be detected reliably by colposcopy and cytology (Figs. 6.113, 6.114, and 6.116). Conservative management is more difficult if the apex of the cone is involved. In this setting, follow-up cytology should be complemented by endocervical curettage. The most difficult cases are those in which the stromal interface is concerned, with the margins running close to or through dysplastic epithelium in endocervical crypts (Figs. 3.21 and 3.23). As with destructive methods, malignant epithelium can be buried in residual crypts after healing and re-epithelialization of the surface. Such cases can be detected with cytology and colposcopy only when they have become invasive and broken through the surface. This also applies to invasive nests close to the resection margins; similar foci can remain in the residual cervix.

Preservation of the uterus must be weighed against the risks. The risk of expectant therapy for patients with incompletely excised superficial lesions is not high, provided regular follow-up is ensured. We have reported on a series of 390 patients with positive margins after cold-knife conization for HSIL. After a mean of 19 years, 78% of patients remained free of disease and 22% had persisting or recurrent CIN 3.

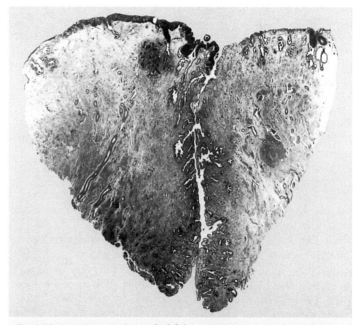

Fig. 3.23 Conization specimen. The left lip contains a microinvasive carcinoma, which shows no connection with the surface epithelium. It measures 3 mm in diameter, and reaches 6 mm in depth. This lesion can be seen with the naked eye in histologic sections. The surface and some crypts show carcinoma in situ (CIN 3, HSIL), extending beyond the external os on the left.

Repeat Conization

Residual lesions after conization can be removed completely with repeat conization, provided there is still sufficient cervical tissue. The technique is the same as for primary conization.

Primary Hysterectomy

The considerations that apply to ablative methods also apply to hysterectomy as the initial treatment of SIL (CIN). Specifically, invasive disease must not be overlooked. Mortality from cervical cancer after primary hysterectomy for presumed intraepithelial neoplasia can be explained only by inadequate diagnosis before the operation. However, not infrequently, patients with SIL have other indications for hysterectomy (e.g., abnormal bleeding, symptomatic fibroids).

Primary hysterectomy should be based on firm indications. The vaginal approach appears indicated because the cervix can be circumcised under direct vision after iodine staining (Schiller's test) for precise delineation of the SIL. Recurrence rates appear lower after vaginal than after abdominal hysterectomy.

Primary Medical Treatment of SIL

Local imiquimod has been used for the treatment of HSIL. This appears a promising option, particularly for younger women with fertility concerns and easily visible lesions on the ectocervix. Studies looking at the potential role of imiquimod and other substances in the treatment of SIL are underway.

3.4.3 Treatment of Microinvasive Carcinoma

The treatment of microinvasive carcinoma (FIGO stage IA) has been as controversial as its definition, for both squamous cell and glandular lesions. In recent decades, the trend has clearly been toward less radical surgery. Most patients can probably be treated with conization alone provided that margins are clear. Controversy persists particularly as to the indications for lymphadenectomy and resection of parametrial tissue. The difficulty lies in selecting patients who need more extensive surgery (i.e., lymphadenectomy, parametrial resection).

Lymphatic space involvement and poor differentiation (confluent growth pattern) appear to be risk factors for recurrence, but considering how common these perceived risk factors are in patients free of recurrence, it is clear that their specificity is low. This supports the view that radical treatment of microinvasive carcinoma is almost always overtreatment.

Less than 2% of such patients have died of carcinoma. Clearly, treatment needs to be individualized. Lymphadenectomy is indicated for patients with extensive vascular space involvement and a poorly differentiated lesion, but removal of parametrial tissue appears unnecessary.

3.4.4 Follow-up after Treatment

Follow-up after treatment consists of colposcopy, cytology, and HPV testing. In women who test negative for HR-HPV at 6 and 24 months posttreatment, the risk of disease seems to be similar to that of the general population. Recurrences after treatment are higher for older than for younger women. The lower recurrence rates in younger women suggest that age-specific immunity may also contribute to the cure of cervical precancer. However, large epidemiologic studies report that the risk of developing or dying from invasive cervical or vaginal cancer in women with a history of treatment for HSIL is two to three times higher than in the general population. This makes clear that women who have been treated for HSIL or AIS require careful surveillance.

Further Reading

Arbyn M, Kyrgiou M, Gondry J, Petry KU, Paraskevaidis E. Long term outcomes for women treated for cervical precancer. BMJ 2014;348:f7700

Batista CS, Atallah AN, Saconato H, da Silva EMK. 5-FU for genital warts in non-immunocompromised individuals. Cochrane Database Syst Rev 2010;4(4):CD006562

Burghardt E, Girardi F, Lahousen M, Pickel H, Tamussino K. Microinvasive carcinoma of the uterine cervix (International Federation of Gynecology and Obstetrics stage IA). Cancer 1991;67(4):1037–1045

Chan BKS, Melnikow J, Slee CA, Arellanes R, Sawaya GF. Posttreatment human papillomavirus testing for recurrent cervical intraepithelial neoplasia: a systematic review. Am J Obstet Gynecol 2009;200(4):422.e1–422.e9

European Federation for Colposcopy and Pathology of the Lower Genital Tract. www.e-f-c.org

Ghaem-Maghami S, Sagi S, Majeed G, Soutter WP. Incomplete excision of cervical intraepithelial neoplasia and risk of treatment failure: a meta-analysis. Lancet Oncol 2007;8(11):985–993

Girardi F, Burghardt E, Pickel H. Small FIGO stage IB cervical cancer. Gynecol Oncol 1994;55(3, Pt 1):427–432

Grimm C, Polterauer S, Natter C, et al. Treatment of cervical intraepithelial neoplasia with topical imiquimod: a randomized controlled trial. Obstet Gynecol 2012;120(1):152–159

Kocken M, Helmerhorst TJ, Berkhof J, et al. Risk of recurrent high-grade cervical intraepithelial neoplasia after successful treatment: a long-term multi-cohort study. Lancet Oncol 2011;12(5):441–450

Manchanda R, Baldwin P, Crawford R, et al. Effect of margin status on cervical intraepithelial neoplasia recurrence following LLETZ in women over 50 years. BJOG 2008;115(10):1238–1242

Martin-Hirsch PP, Paraskevaidis E, Bryant A, Dickinson HO. Surgery for cervical intraepithelial neoplasia. Cochrane Database Syst Rev 2013;12(12):CD001318

Melnikow J, McGahan C, Sawaya GF, Ehlen T, Coldman A. Cervical intraepithelial neoplasia outcomes after treatment: long-term follow-up from the British Columbia Cohort Study. J Natl Cancer Inst 2009;101(10):721–728

Reich O, Lahousen M, Pickel H, Tamussino K, Winter R. Cervical intraepithelial neoplasia III: long-term follow-up after cold-knife conization with involved margins. Obstet Gynecol 2002;99(2):193–196

Reich O, Pickel H, Lahousen M, Tamussino K, Winter R. Cervical intraepithelial neoplasia III: long-term outcome after cold-knife conization with clear margins. Obstet Gynecol 2001;97(3):428–430

Reich O, Pickel H, Tamussino K, Winter R. Microinvasive carcinoma of the cervix: site of first focus of invasion. Obstet Gynecol 2001;97(6):890–892

Schiller W. Early diagnosis of carcinoma of the cervix. Surg Gynecol Obstet 1933;56:210–222

Strander B, Hällgren J, Sparén P. Effect of ageing on cervical or vaginal cancer in Swedish women previously treated for cervical intraepithelial neoplasia grade 3: population based cohort study of long term incidence and mortality. BMJ 2014;348:f7361

Chapter 4

Teaching and Training Colposcopy

4

4 Teaching and Training Colposcopy

The colposcope itself is a simple instrument, even for beginners. The eyepieces are adjusted individually. The instrument is focused by moving the swivel arm to the working distance for the particular scope. It is usually unnecessary to use the fine focus. Magnification × 10 is quite adequate for routine work; higher magnification is needed only to study details. Smaller enlargements can be used for imaging the entire cervix. Colpophotography is straightforward and produces high-quality pictures. The cervix has to be well exposed and the camera focused.

Although the colposcope is straightforward to use, proficiency in colposcopy requires a knowledge of colposcopic concepts and an appreciation of cervical pathology. Once a working knowledge of colposcopic findings has been acquired from a textbook, atlas, or teaching slides, it is helpful to work with an experienced colposcopist who can demonstrate and explain the exam and findings. Obtaining a biopsy should be demonstrated and then practiced. Courses where individual problems can be discussed with the faculty are available at entry and advanced levels.

Video systems are very helpful for teaching colposcopy. Video nicely shows the dynamics of changes after application of acetic acid and iodine. Video also lets the patient follow the examination.

Improvement takes practice. We use the colposcope at every speculum examination. By doing this, the practitioner gains an easy routine and does not find colposcopy unnecessarily time-consuming. Routine colposcopy expedites the appreciation of benign findings in women of all ages, and familiarity with benign findings makes one more alert to those that are no longer benign. It is logical to start with the study of ectopy and continue with the protean manifestations of the transformation zone. We believe this approach fosters an understanding of the dynamics of the events at the cervix, which, if they take a wrong turn, can lead to atypia and neoplasia.

Certain colposcopic findings are easy to categorize either as benign or as highly suspicious, but in between there is a wide spectrum of appearances that can be challenging to interpret. The same applies to cytology. The degree of confidence depends on the examiner's skill and experience. Biopsying questionable findings is part of the learning curve and avoids serious mistakes. By correlating colposcopic findings with histologic findings, the practitioner will gain confidence and take fewer biopsies. The chance of missing a significant finding is considerably reduced by concomitant cytology and human papillomavirus testing.

In recent years, there have been national and international efforts to improve and standardize training in colposcopy.

4.1 Colposcopy Training in Europe

Colposcopy plays a pivotal role in cervical cancer screening. It enables treatment of premalignant lesions, but, of equal importance, it prevents needless intervention. Cervical screening saves lives, but the vast majority of women screened are well and would never develop cervical cancer. It is axiomatic that there is potential for harm. Treating all women with abnormal smears would prevent the development of cervical cancers, but this would be at great cost. Colposcopy is therefore primarily about selection.

Colposcopic performance depends on the observer as well as on the clinical context in which the examination takes place. As noted earlier, the authors of this book recommend routine colposcopy as part of the gynecologic examination. While certainly good for experience, this approach is not feasible in all settings. Colposcopic findings are subjective and the related management decisions require problem-solving skills and experience. A colposcopist needs diagnostic and management skills, which necessitate both adequate training and a sufficient workload to maintain skills.

The indications for colposcopy vary from country to country due to differences in health care models, but its core objective is the same, namely, to detect preinvasive cervical changes so as to allow treatment and thereby prevent the development of invasive cancer. The International Federation of Cervical Pathology and Colposcopy (IFCPC) and the European Federation for Colposcopy (EFC) have recognized that adequate training was the key to ensuring high-quality colposcopy.

4.1.1 Developing European Standards in Colposcopy Training

Despite the self-evident value of sharing common standards for training throughout Europe, the task of achieving such a goal is challenging. In part, this is due to the different models of health care and medical training in different countries. The strength of the EFC is that it is a federation of national societies that can collectively reach a consensus, and the individual societies can then deliver the agreed initiatives in a way that is relevant to their country. The following summarizes the EFC guidelines for training in colposcopy that have been developed over the years. While programs may contain theoretical or practical courses, colposcopic training requires apprenticeship-type experience. Colposcopists need to acquire a range of professional skills in addition to diagnostic ability. Training programs should include all of the following areas.

Development of Clinical Competence

A training program requires a curriculum, structure, and trainers. The EFC identified the core competencies needed to undertake diagnostic colposcopy and, where applicable, to undertake therapeutic procedures. A core curriculum was developed that now forms the basis of the syllabi for many European national societies, including Spain, Germany, and the United Kingdom.

The training program is focused on transferring theoretical knowledge into practical performance. The EFC advises that the trainee perform at least 150 colposcopies under supervision. Clinical experience is based on direct clinical supervision (50 cases) and indirect clinical supervision (100 cases). All cases should be discussed and reviewed. Ideally, the best time for this feedback is at the end of each training session.

A structured apprenticeship approach avoids the danger of the required training becoming overloaded with extraneous and irrelevant items. Most trainees would already have a significant knowledge base prior to training, and it would be redundant to revise the associated disciplines of cytology, histology, and pathology in isolation from the knowledge they require in order to practice competently. This methodology is relevant and reflects real-life clinical practice. The "on-the-job" nature of the program makes learning more effective, as knowledge is not being acquired in isolation. The syllabus details a number of competencies in the logbook that the trainee needs to acquire.

Electronic Logbook

A logbook is a convenient and effective way of documenting progression through training as well as a detailed record of all the cases seen. The logbook records clinical experience and is reviewed by the trainer periodically to assess experience and to overview the correlation between colposcopic findings and histology. The EFC has produced an electronic logbook, which can be accessed via the British Society for Colposcopy and Cervical Pathology (BSCCP) website (www.bsccp.org.uk). As per EFC guidelines, the logbook documents the requirements of 50 cases performed under direct and 100 cases performed under indirect supervision.

Assessment and Exit Examination

The training syllabus is detailed in the logbook. The responsibility of ensuring that it is adequately covered and the relevant experience gained lies with the trainee. The trainer helps the trainee to learn through discussion and provides advice not only on their diagnostic technique but also on case management. There are a variety of educational tools that can be used in assessments. They are typically structured processes that variously can assess surgical skill, aspects of clinical activity, or behavior. The EFC recommends that training programs should have a form of summative exit assessment.

4.2 European Diploma in Colposcopy

The EFC aims to promote uniformly high-quality colposcopy throughout Europe, and there is a proposition to develop a European qualification in colposcopy (Table 4.1). The goal is to promote uniform training to raise clinical standards, and that training in one country might be recognized in another. Realizing this aspiration will require training programs to be harmonized, with a common curriculum and quality assurance. While these measures seem remote at present, it is evident that the EFC has enabled significant steps toward this goal.

Table 4.1 EFC core competencies for colposcopic training

General training
Understand the development of cervical neoplasia
Ensure that practice complies with health and safety recommendations
Manage patients within EFC guidelines
Provide adequate information prior to colposcopy
Answer questions about management
Communicate with other health professionals
Understand national cervical screening guidelines
Be able to communicate results in a sensitive manner
Provide data to a national body
Basic examination
Be able to take a history
Examine the vagina
Examine the vulva
Position and adjust the colposcope
Be able to position a patient for colposcopy
Be able to insert a vaginal speculum
Use endocervical speculum
Document colposcopic findings
Provide adequate information after colposcopy
Colposcopic procedure
Perform cervical sampling (including cytobrush)
Perform bacteriologic swabs
Examine the transformation zone with acetic acid
Perform Schiller's iodine test
Examine the transformation zone with saline and green filter
Quantify and describe acetic acid changes
Colposcopic findings
Determine whether colposcopy is satisfactory or not
Determine the type of transformation zone (1,2,3)
Recognize the extent of abnormal epithelium
Recognize original squamous epithelium
Recognize columnar epithelium
Recognize metaplastic epithelium
Recognize congenital transformation zone
Recognize minor colposcopic changes
Recognize major colposcopic changes
Recognize features suggestive of invasion
Recognize abnormal vascular patterns
Recognize changes associated with previous treatment
Recognize the effects of pregnancy on the cervix
Recognize acute inflammatory changes
Recognize VAIN
Recognize VIN
Recognize benign cervical polyps
Recognize condyloma plana
Recognize condylomata acuminata
Biopsies and treatment
Obtain informed consent for performing a procedure
Be able to administer local analgesia
Determine where to take directed biopsies
Perform directed vaginal biopsies
Perform directed vulvar biopsies
Control bleeding from biopsy sites

Abbreviations: EFC, European Federation for Colposcopy; VAIN, vaginal intraepithelial neoplasia; VIN, vulvar intraepithelial neoplasia.

Further Reading

European Federation for Colposcopy and Pathology of the Lower Genital Tract. Available at: www.e-f-c.org

International Federation of Cervical Pathology and Colposcopy (IFCPC). Available at: http://www.ifcpc.org/en/education

Moss EL, Redman CWE, Arbyn M, et al. Colposcopy training and assessment across the member countries of the European Federation for Colposcopy. Eur J Obstet Gynecol Reprod Biol 2015;188:124–128

Redman CWE, Dollery E, Jordan JA. Development of the European colposcopy core curriculum: use of the Delphi technique. J Obstet Gynaecol 2004;24(7):780–784

Redman C, Jordan J. How can the European Federation for Colposcopy promote high quality colposcopy throughout Europe? Coll Antropol 2007;31(Suppl 2):131–133

Shehmar M, Cruikshank M, Finn C, Redman C, Fraser I, Peile E. A validity study of the national UK colposcopy objective structured clinical examination—is it a test fit for purpose? BJOG 2009;116(13):1796–1799, discussion 1799–1800

Chapter 5

Colposcopic Terminology

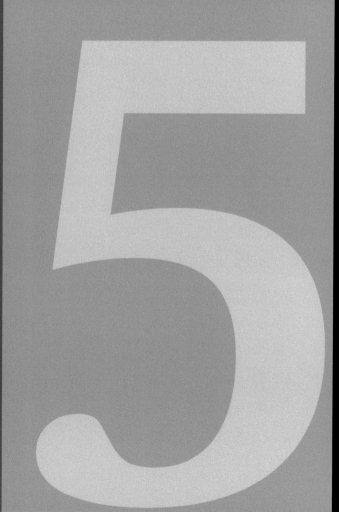

5 Colposcopic Terminology

The latest version of the international terminology, which is used in this book, was formulated by the International Federation of Cervical Pathology and Colposcopy (IFCPC) with the International Society for the Study of Vulvar Disease (ISSVD) in Rio de Janeiro, Brazil, in 2011. This current version provides a comprehensive terminology for the entire lower genital tract and thus includes vulvar, vaginal, and anal disease as well as cervical findings. It also specifies terminology for different excision techniques and excision specimen dimensions (Tables 5.1–5.5).

Table 5.1 2011 International Federation for Cervical Pathology and Colposcopy colposcopic terminology of the cervix

General assessment		Adequate/inadequate for the reason (e.g., cervix obscured by inflammation, bleeding, scar)	
		SCJ visibility: completely visible, partially visible, not visible	
		TZ types 1, 2, 3	
Normal colposcopic findings		Original squamous epithelium:	
		Mature	
		Atrophic	
		Columnar epithelium	
		Ectopy	
		Metaplastic squamous epithelium	
		Nabothian cysts	
		Crypt (gland) openings	
		Deciduosis in pregnancy	
Abnormal colposcopic findings	General principles	Location of the lesion:	
		Inside or outside the TZ	
		By clock position	
		Size of the lesion:	
		Number of cervical quadrants the lesion covers	
		Size as percentage of cervix	
	Grade 1 (minor)	Thin acetowhite epithelium	Fine mosaic, fine punctation
		Irregular, geographic border	
	Grade 2 (major)	Dense acetowhite epithelium, rapid appearance of acetowhitening, cuffed crypt (gland) openings	Coarse mosaic, coarse punctation, sharp border, inner border sign, ridge sign
	Nonspecific	Leukoplakia (keratosis, hyperkeratosis), erosion, Lugol's staining (Schiller's test): stained/nonstained	
Suspicious for invasion		Atypical vessels	
		Additional signs: fragile vessels, irregular surface, exophytic lesion, necrosis, ulceration (necrotic), tumor/gross neoplasm	
Miscellaneous findings		Congenital TZ, condyloma, polyp (ectocervical/endocervical), inflammation	Stenosis, congenital anomaly, post-treatment consequence, endometriosis

Abbreviations: SCJ, squamocolumnar junction; TZ, transformation zone.

Table 5.2 International Federation for Cervical Pathology and Colposcopy definitions of excision types and dimensions of cone specimens

Excision treatment types	
Type 1	Resection of a completely ectocervical or type 1 TZ
Type 2	Resection of a type 2 TZ (small amount of endocervical epithelium visible with a colposcope)
Type 3	Resection of a type 3 TZ (longer and larger amount of tissue than type 1 or type 2 excisions, with a significant amount of endocervical epithelium)
Excision specimen dimensions	Length: distance from the distal or external margin to the proximal or internal margin
	Thickness: distance from the stromal margin to the surface of the excised specimen
	Circumference (optional): perimeter of the excised specimen

Abbreviation: TZ, transformation zone.

Table 5.3 2011 International Federation for Cervical Pathology and Colposcopy clinical/colposcopic terminology of the vagina

General assessment	Adequate/inadequate for the reason (e.g., inflammation, bleeding, scar)	
Normal colposcopic findings	Squamous epithelium:	
	Mature	
	Atrophic	
Abnormal colposcopic findings	General principles	Upper one-third/lower two-thirds, anterior/posterior/lateral (right or left)
	Grade 1 (minor)	Thin acetowhite epithelium, fine punctation fine mosaic
	Grade 2 (major)	Dense acetowhite epithelium, coarse punctation coarse mosaic
	Suspicious for invasion	Atypical vessels
		Additional signs: fragile vessels, irregular surface, exophytic lesion, necrosis, ulceration (necrotic), tumor/gross neoplasm
	Nonspecific	Columnar epithelium (adenosis); Lesion staining by Lugol's solution (Schiller's test): stained/nonstained, leukoplakia
Miscellaneous findings		Erosion (traumatic), condyloma, polyp, cyst, endometriosis, inflammation, vaginal stenosis, congenital transformation zone

Table 5.4 2011 International Federation for Cervical Pathology and Colposcopy clinical/colposcopic terminology of the vulva (including the anus)

Section		Pattern
Basic definitions	Various structures: Urethra, Skene's duct openings, clitoris, prepuce, frenulum, mons pubis, labia minora, labia majora, interlabial sulci, vestibule, vestibular duct openings, Bartholin's duct openings, hymen, fourchette, perineum, anus, anal SCJ (dentate line)	Composition: Squamous epithelium—hairy/nonhairy, mucosa
Normal findings		Micropapillomatosis, sebaceous glands (Fordyce's spots), vestibular redness
Abnormal findings	General principles: Size in centimeters, location	Lesion type: Macule, patch, papule, plaque nodule, cyst, vesicle, bulla, pustule Lesion color: Skin-colored, red, white, dark Secondary morphology: Eczema, lichenification, excoriation, purpura, scarring, ulcer, erosion, fissure, wart
	Abnormal colposcopic or other magnification findings	Acetowhite epithelium, punctation, atypical vessels, surface irregularities, abnormal anal SCJ (note location about dentate line)
Suspicion of malignancy	With or without white, gray, red or brown discoloration	Gross neoplasm, ulceration, necrosis, bleeding, exophytic lesion, hyperkeratosis
Miscellaneous findings		Trauma, malformation

Abbreviation: SCJ, squamocolumnar junction.

Table 5.5 Definitions of primary lesion types of the vulva

Term	Definition
Macule	Small (<1.5 cm) area of color change; no elevation and no substance of palpation
Patch	Large (>1.5 cm) area of color change; no elevation and no substance of palpation
Papule	Small (<1.5 cm) elevated and palpable lesion
Plaque	Large (>1.5 cm) elevated, palpable, and flat-topped lesion
Nodule	Large (>1.5 cm) often hemispherical or poorly marginated; may be located on the surface, within or below the skin; nodules may be cystic or solid
Vesicle	Small (<1.5 cm) fluid-filled blister; the fluid is clear (blister: a compartmentalized, fluid-filled elevation of the skin or mucosa)
Bulla	Large (>1.5 cm) fluid-filled blister; the fluid is clear
Pustule	Pus-filled blister; the fluid is white or yellow

Further Reading

Bornstein J, Bentley J, Bösze P, et al. 2011 colposcopic terminology of the International Federation for Cervical Pathology and Colposcopy. Obstet Gynecol 2012;120(1):166–172

Bornstein J, Sideri M, Tatti S, Walker P, Prendiville W, Haefner HK; Nomenclature Committee of International Federation for Cervical Pathology and Colposcopy. 2011 terminology of the vulva of the International Federation for Cervical Pathology and Colposcopy. J Low Genit Tract Dis 2012;16(3):290–295

Nayar R, Wilbur D. The Bethesda System for Reporting Cervical Cytology. New York: Springer; 2015

Chapter 6

Colposcopic Findings

6 Colposcopic Findings

It is important to appreciate that very similar colposcopic appearance can be produced by different biologic processes. Understanding this requires knowledge of the underlying histology. The relationship between cervical histology and pathology and colposcopic diagnosis is fundamental and reciprocal.

6.1 Normal Colposcopic Appearances

6.1.1 Original Squamous Epithelium

Like other normal superficial squamous epithelia, the native, original squamous epithelium of the uterine cervix is smooth and uninterrupted by gland openings (Fig. 6.1). This sets it apart from normal squamous epithelium that has arisen through metaplasia. More detailed observation of a surface covered by epithelium of metaplastic origin shows gland (crypt) openings and retention cysts, which indicate that the area was originally occupied by columnar epithelium (Figs. 6.2 and 6.3a–c). The original squamous epithelium during the reproductive period displays a reddish color that can vary from pale to intense pink during the various phases of the menstrual cycle. It stains deep brown with iodine, reflecting its glycogen content (Fig. 6.3c).

The so-called portio rugata is seen especially during adolescence. The cervix is dome-shaped, with a dimple-like os but can expand distally to resemble a mushroom (Fig. 6.4). Sometimes the surface looks like a cockscomb (Fig. 6.5a, b). This is probably an incidental finding without clinical relevance.

6.1.2 Atrophic Squamous Epithelium

After menopause, in the absence of estrogen, the squamous epithelium becomes thin and devoid of glycogen, and the stromal blood supply diminishes. These changes result in a pale epithelium that can show a fine network of capillaries (Fig. 6.6a). The epithelial thinning and loss of glycogen are patchy, resulting in a stippled appearance with iodine because of its irregular uptake (Fig. 6.6b). In older women, the epithelium assumes a uniform light brown to yellow color as a result of complete loss of glycogen (Fig. 6.7). The thin epithelial covering is fragile and makes the terminal vessels vulnerable to minor trauma, which can result in erosions and subepithelial hemorrhages (Fig. 6.8).

6.1.3 Ectopy (Columnar Epithelium)

Ideally, the original squamocolumnar junction (SCJ) is situated at the external os. Depending on the size, shape, and patulosity of the external os, varying portions of the canal may be visible. In patulous cervices, the architecture of endocervical mucosa can be seen clearly (Fig. 6.9).

In adolescents and young women, the columnar epithelium is frequently situated on the ectocervix at some distance from the external os. This is referred to as *ectopy*. In cases of marked eversion of the endocervical mucosa, its rugose architecture becomes evident (Figs. 6.10–6.12a, b).

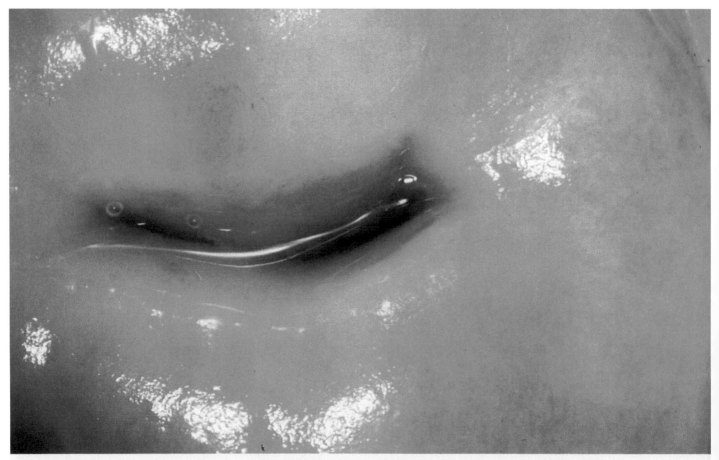

Fig. 6.1 Original squamous epithelium in a woman of reproductive age. The surface is completely smooth and displays a fresh reddish color.

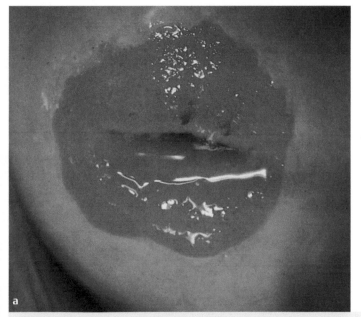 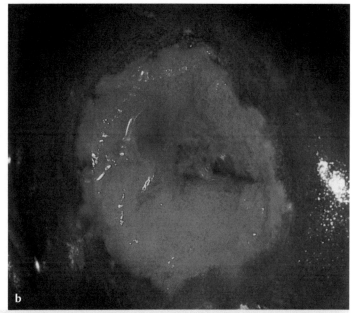

Fig. 6.2 (a) Ectopy before application of acetic acid. The gland openings at the 10 o'clock position indicate earlier transformation. **(b)** After application of iodine. The columnar epithelium does not stain; it is merely discolored by the thin film covering it. The demarcation from the deep brown original squamous epithelium is indistinct.

Ectopy appears classically as a "red patch" (Fig. 6.2a). Grossly, it may look suspicious to the inexperienced examiner. More detailed colposcopic examination shows its unique papillary architecture, which identifies its real nature. Ectopy does not stain with iodine (Fig. 6.2b).

Ectopy is usually covered by mucus secreted by the columnar epithelium. Acetic acid helps to remove the mucus (see Chapter 3), revealing the distinctive papillary structure. Acetic acid also causes the tissue to swell, throwing the mucosal architecture into sharp relief and giving the papillae a grapelike appearance. The intense red of the red patch changes to pink or whitish (Figs. 6.3 and 6.13).

The SCJ is usually sharp and step-like (Figs. 6.2, 6.9, and 6.13). Careful inspection often reveals a slender, white margin and gland openings, which indicates the initiation of transformation (Figs. 6.3, 6.11, and 6.14). It is important to pay close attention to the margins of ectopy so as not to overlook significant colposcopic lesions.

Ectopic columnar epithelium is less resilient and more vulnerable to trauma than squamous epithelium. It is subject to contact bleeding at speculum examination (contact bleeding should also make the examiner consider the possibility of cancer). Although neoplastic papillary fronds tend to be coarse and irregular, they can be mistaken for benign changes.

The influence of exogenous and endogenous sex steroids on the transformation of the columnar epithelium has been studied longitudinally (Fig. 6.15a–d). Estrogen-containing oral contraceptives appear to have a positive and enhancing effect on ectopy, and women who discontinue contraceptives show transformation in a relatively brief time (Fig. 6.16a, b).

6.1.4 Transformation Zone

The transformation zone (TZ) can appear as a nonspecific red area. Sometimes there is a fine vascular pattern (Fig. 6.17a). Application of acetic acid turns the previously red epithelium grayish white. Within the TZ are openings of cervical glands (crypts) and small islands of residual columnar epithelium. The demarcation from the original squamous epithelium is indistinct (Fig. 6.17b).

The process of transformation characteristically begins at the SCJ. The flat epithelial margin around the periphery of an ectopy can be distinguished from the original squamous as well as columnar epithelium by its variable color and by the presence of gland openings (Figs. 6.2, 6.6, and 6.18–6.20).

The surface contour of an ectopy changes as transformation takes place. The papillae become coarse and fused, resulting in only slight fissuring of the surface. These changes signify the initiation of squamous metaplasia. Fields of metaplastic epithelium within a TZ may vary widely in their maturation, easily verifiable by application of iodine (the Schiller's test), which is a sensitive indicator of epithelial maturity (Fig. 6.20b).

The topographic progression of transformation can be haphazard, and its stage of development can vary markedly from one part of the periphery to another. Islands of squamous epithelium can appear in a sea of columnar epithelium; these must have arisen by metaplasia (Figs. 6.15a–d, 6.16a, b, and 6.19). The metaplastic epithelium can form tongues or fingerlike processes that interdigitate with intact columnar epithelium (Fig. 6.21). Even when most of an ectopy is fully transformed, small islands of columnar epithelium can remain; this appearance is referred to as *TZ with ectopic residuals* (Fig. 6.22). Longitudinal study of the TZ over years is particularly informative (Figs. 6.15 and 6.16).

The transformation of an ectopy from columnar to squamous epithelium does not always proceed to completion. Areas of the newly formed squamous epithelium can be fully mature, whereas other parts of an ectopy can remain columnar for long periods (Fig. 6.23). The new SCJ is again situated at the external os. Squamous epithelium of metaplastic origin can be distinguished from original squamous epithelium by the presence of gland openings, more prominent vessels (Fig. 6.24), or retention cysts (Fig. 6.25). Undulations from numerous retention cysts (nabothian follicles), with long vessels coursing over their surface, are also characteristic (Fig. 6.26). The vasculature in such cases is so typical that the presence of deep-seated and otherwise invisible cysts can be easily inferred (Figs. 6.132 and 6.133).

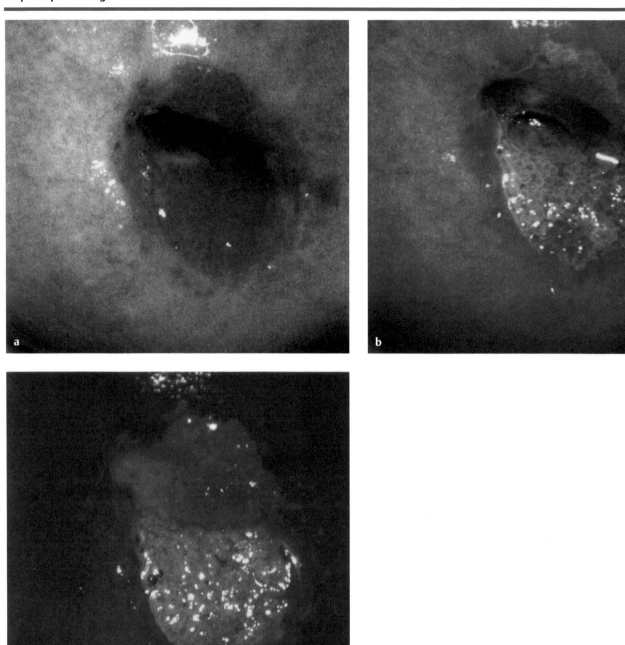

Fig. 6.3 Small red area on the anterior and posterior lip of the external os. **(a)** Before application of acetic acid. **(b)** After application of 3% acetic acid. **(c)** After application of iodine. The columnar epithelium does not stain. The transformation zone at the margins is identifiable by the incomplete staining of the new squamous cell epithelium.

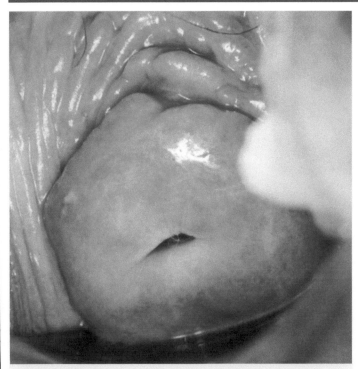

Fig. 6.4 The portio rugata in a 29-year-old woman. Squamocolumnar junction not visible (type III transformation zone). (This image is provided courtesy of O. Baader.)

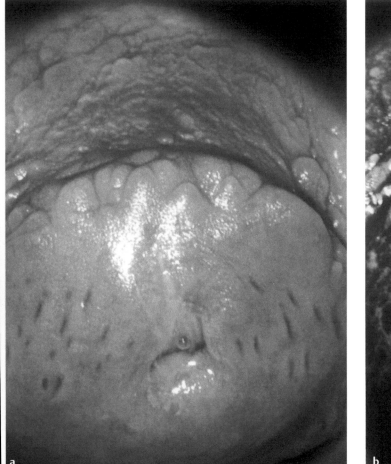

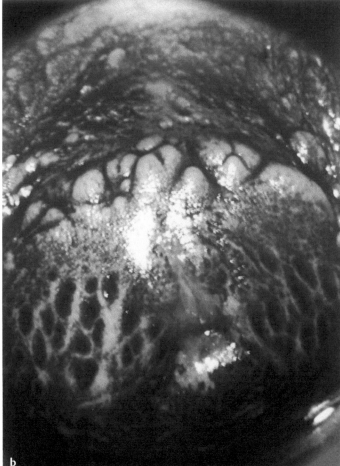

Fig. 6.5 (a) Original squamous epithelium. Cockscomb-like lesion on the anterior lip and fornix in a 17-year-old girl. The polypoid contour around the external os is suggested only by the shallow notches. **(b)** Surprising stippling effect of iodine. Only the posterior lip shows typical uniform mahogany-brown staining. (This image is provided courtesy of O. Baader.)

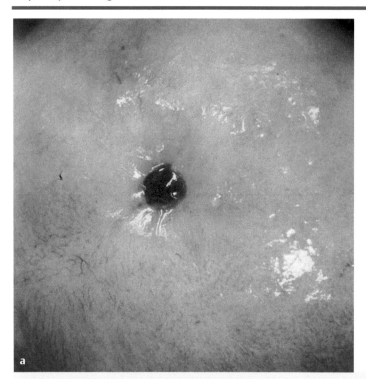

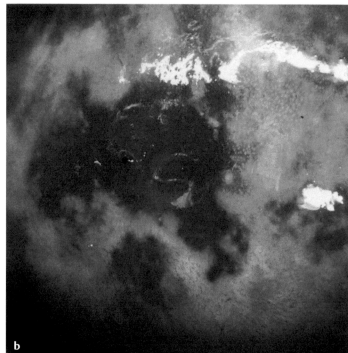

Fig. 6.6 **(a)** Atrophic squamous epithelium in a postmenopausal woman. Fine blood vessels shine through the thin epithelium, which appears pale pink to yellowish. **(b)** The same cervix after application of iodine. The characteristic stippled appearance is due to focal glycogen retention.

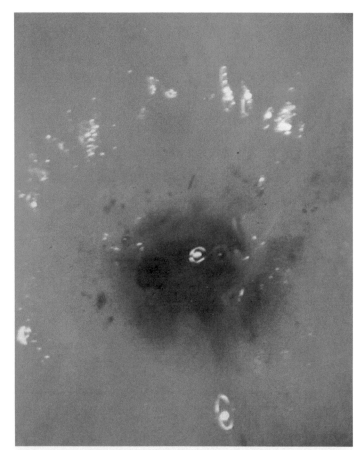

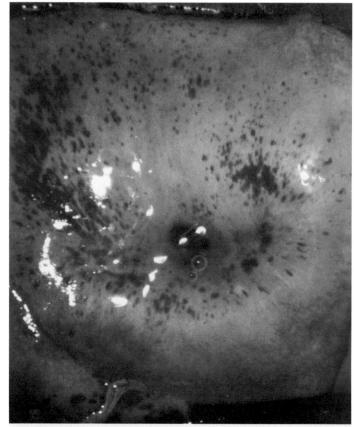

Fig. 6.7 The loss of glycogen is uniform in the atrophic epithelium of an older woman, resulting in homogeneous yellow staining with iodine.

Fig. 6.8 With advancing age, the squamous epithelium becomes fragile. Subepithelial hemorrhages may appear during vaginal examination. Note the fine vessels that run toward the os.

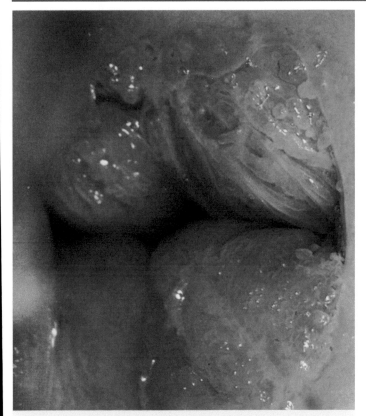

Fig. 6.9 The original squamocolumnar junction of this gaping cervix is most distinct. The anterior lip displays a thin rim of transformation zone. The rugose structure of the endocervical mucosa is clearly seen.

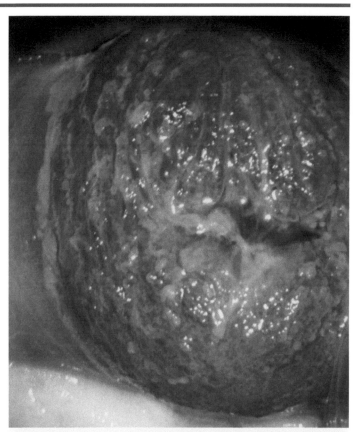

Fig. 6.10 Eversion of the endocervical mucosa (ectopy), with its rugose architecture thrown into sharp relief.

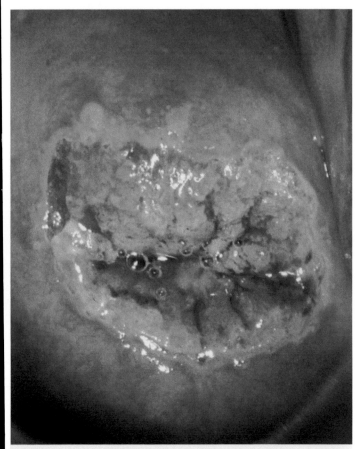

Fig. 6.11 Apparent eversion (ectopy) of a cervix with a patulous os resulting from wide separation of the speculum. A thin rim of transformation zone is visible near the junction with the original squamous epithelium.

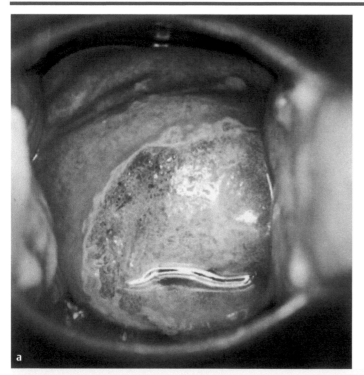

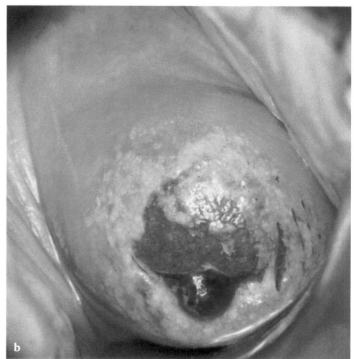

Fig. 6.12 (a) Ectopy with a thin rim of transformation zone (TZ) in a 14-year-old. **(b)** After 2 years, the transformation is more advanced. Squamocolumnar junction fully visible (type 1 TZ). (This image is provided courtesy of O. Baader.)

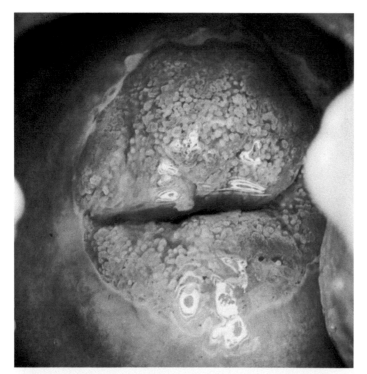

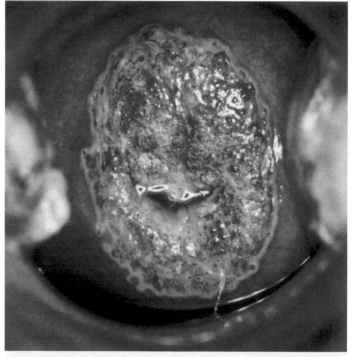

Fig. 6.13 Typical appearance of ectopy after application of acetic acid. The grapelike structure is unmistakable. Note the whitish rim of transformation zone at the periphery.

Fig. 6.14 Ectopy with a slim margin of transformation at the periphery in a 29-year-old nullipara (type 1 transformation zone). (This image is provided courtesy of O. Baader.)

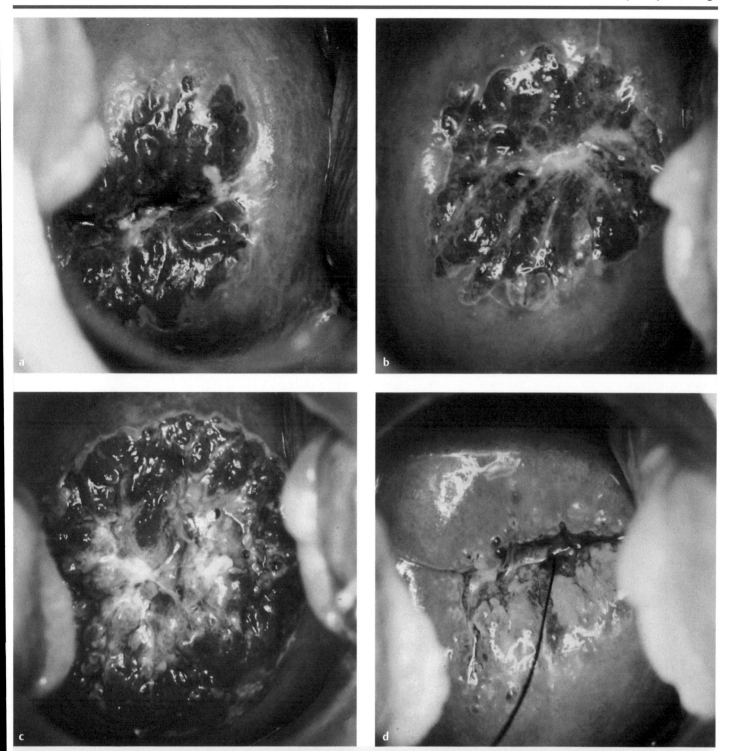

Fig. 6.15 Longitudinal follow-up of a 20-year-old woman beginning oral contraception (OC). **(a)** Before starting OC, there is ectopy with a slim margin of transformation (type 1 transformation zone [TZ]). **(b)** After several months of OC, the ectopy has assumed a strongly coarse papillary appearance. **(c)** At this point, the woman has resumed OC after a vaginal delivery. The ectopy is again apparent. **(d)** The woman received an intrauterine contraceptive device 9 months later and discontinued OC. Three months later, the ectopy has been rapidly transformed (type 1 TZ). (This image is provided courtesy of O. Baader.)

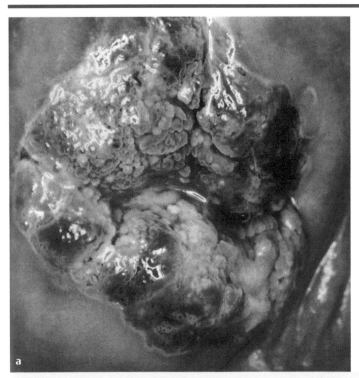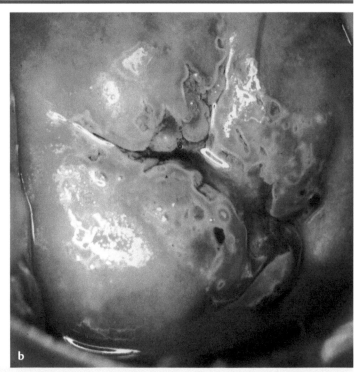

Fig. 6.16 Transformation of marked ectopy with discontinuation of oral contraception (OC). **(a)** Marked ectopy with coarse papillae in a woman with 4 years of OC. **(b)** Only 1 year after discontinued OC (and intrauterine device insertion), there is advanced transformation of the ectopy (type 1 TZ). (This image is provided courtesy of O. Baader.)

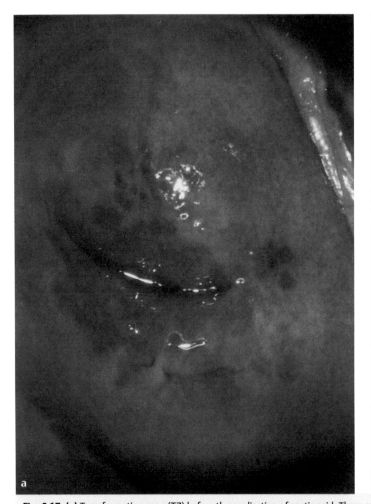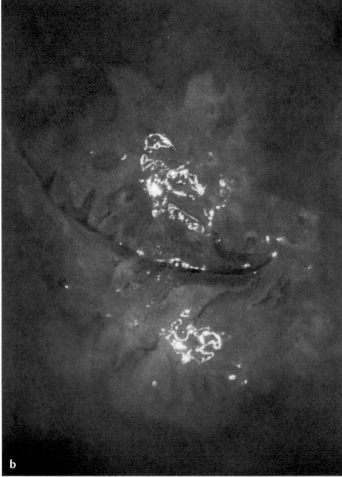

Fig. 6.17 (a) Transformation zone (TZ) before the application of acetic acid. There are small, unremarkable vessels at the edge of the reddish area on the posterior lip of the cervix. **(b)** After application of acetic acid, the previously reddish epithelium is grayish white. Gland openings and small islands of residual columnar epithelium are signs of the TZ.

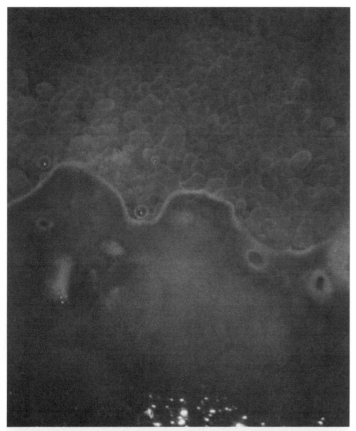

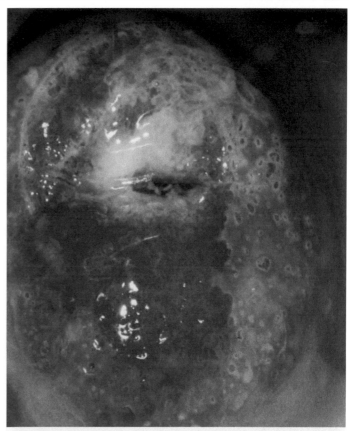

Fig. 6.18 Step-like border between the grapelike structure of the glandular epithelium (ectopy) and the squamous epithelium of the transformation zone. Note the gland openings at the periphery of the squamous epithelium, indicating completed transformation at the edge of the previously larger ectopic area.

Fig. 6.19 Transformation zone. Here, too, the process begins peripherally and spreads toward the center in an irregular manner. Note the smooth surface in spite of the incomplete transformation. There are numerous gland openings.

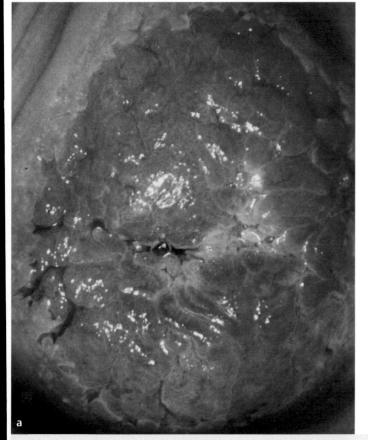

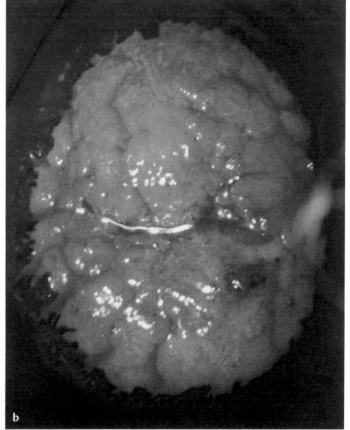

Fig. 6.20 **(a)** Transformation zone. Centrally, within this ectopy, the villi become plumper and fuse to eventually form a flat surface. **(b)** The same patient after application of iodine. The transformed epithelium is mature and contains glycogen. Gland openings are well displayed. The central part does not take up iodine, which merely covers it like a veil.

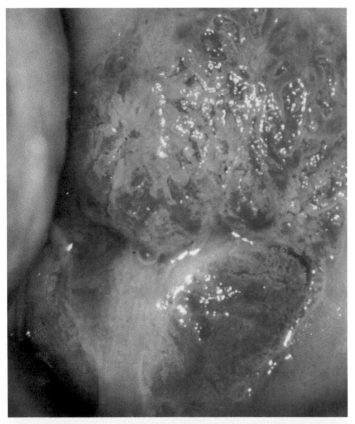

Fig. 6.21 Fingerlike processes of metaplastic epithelium extend centrally from the periphery and interdigitate with islands of columnar epithelium. The transformation involves only the anterior lip.

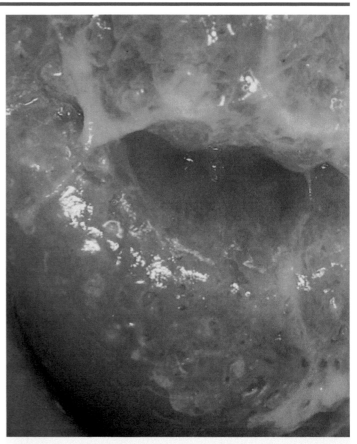

Fig. 6.22 Transformation zone with residual islands of grapelike columnar epithelium on the anterior lip.

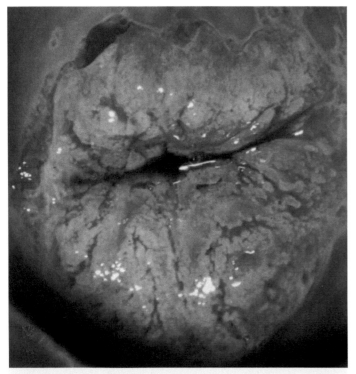

Fig. 6.23 Partial transformation. The transformation zone on the anterior lip takes up only a small portion of the ectopy, which is largely unchanged, apart from enlargement and fusion of its papillae.

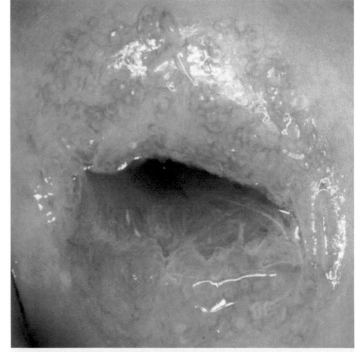

Fig. 6.24 Well-established transformation zone. Although the color of the new squamous epithelium is hardly distinguishable from that of the original, the border of the transformation is marked by fine blood vessels. The new squamocolumnar junction is abrupt.

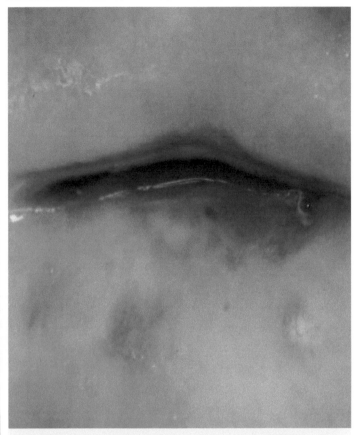

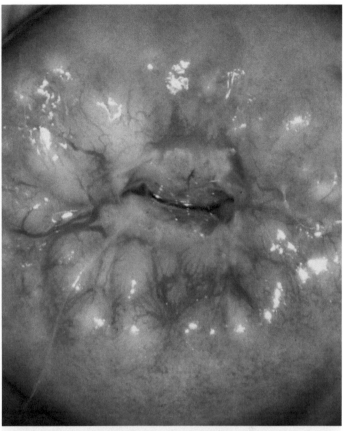

Fig. 6.25 Nabothian follicles covered by smooth squamous epithelium. They are the only indicators of earlier transformation. Blood vessels characteristically run over the surface of the retention cyst on the right.

Fig. 6.26 Nabothian follicles in an established transformation zone. The long, regularly branching blood vessels that shine through the attenuated epithelium are typical.

6.2 Abnormal Colposcopic Findings

6.2.1 Acetowhite Epithelium

The 2011 International Federation for Cervical Pathology and Colposcopy nomenclature distinguishes between *thin* and *dense* acetowhite epithelium, the former being a minor change and the latter a major change. Rapid appearance of acetowhitening is also considered a major change. Acetowhite epithelium does not show mosaic, punctation, or leukoplakia. It does usually contain gland openings and even retention cysts. It usually corresponds to the normal TZ but differs from it in several important aspects. It is characterized by the hallmarks of transformation (e.g., gland openings, retention cysts, residual islands of columnar epithelium) but differs from normal in one or more of the following features:

- A dull to yellow-red color before application of acetic acid.
- A more pronounced color change from red to white with acetic acid application.
- Cuffed gland openings.
- A richer vascularity with occasional atypical vessels.
- A characteristic canary yellow tinge after application of iodine, with at least part of its circumference being sharply demarcated.

These criteria do not always signify the development of atypical epithelium. Transformation can also result in a metaplastic epithelium with only slight keratinization and no elongated stromal papillae and thus will not appear colposcopically as keratosis, punctation, or mosaic. Compared with original squamous epithelium, metaplastic epithelium undergoes a more distinct color change with acetic acid, and its junction with original squamous epithelium is sharply defined (Fig. 6.27). In spite of these differences, it is not always possible to distinguish colposcopically between metaplastic epithelium and squamous intraepithelial lesion (SIL). Even the whitish epithelium of high-grade SIL (HSIL) may be only discrete (thin acetowhite epithelium) so that it can be difficult to distinguish from a normal TZ (Fig. 6.28).

There may be subtle hints of the presence of white epithelium before application of acetic acid. Any shade of red other than the fresh red of the normal TZ should be viewed with suspicion. Grayish red tones, which give the TZ an opaque appearance, and yellow shades, which are probably due to marked inflammatory infiltration of the stroma (Figs. 6.29 and 6.30a), are particularly worrisome. In such cases, acetic acid usually induces a distinct white color change and reveals sharp borders (Figs. 6.29b and 6.30b). A rich vascular bed suggests unusual transformation but is not pathognomonic of epithelial atypia (Fig. 6.31).

The best diagnostic criterion is the acetic acid test. The more marked and the more rapid the color change and the greater the swelling, the greater the likelihood of epithelial atypia (dense acetowhite epithelium; Figs. 6.30b, 6.32, and 6.33). However, the spectrum of color changes is wide (Figs. 6.34 and 6.35a).

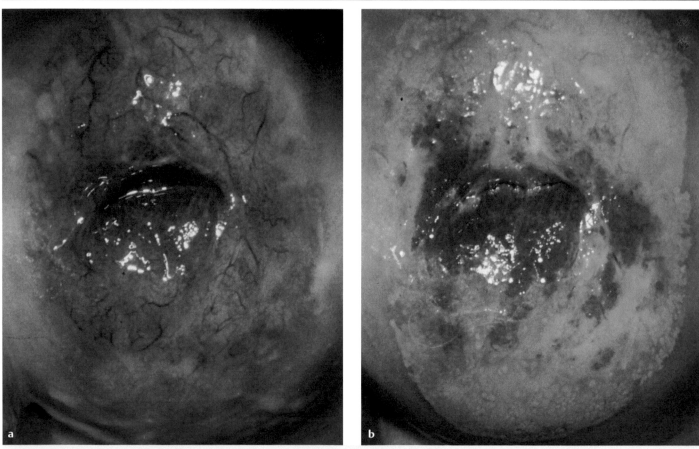

Fig. 6.27 **(a)** Regularly branching blood vessels in a reddish yellow, colposcopically abnormal lesion before application of acetic acid. **(b)** Acetic acid suppresses the vascular pattern but brings out a sharply demarcated fine mosaic with a distinct change in color tone. Histology showed metaplastic epithelium.

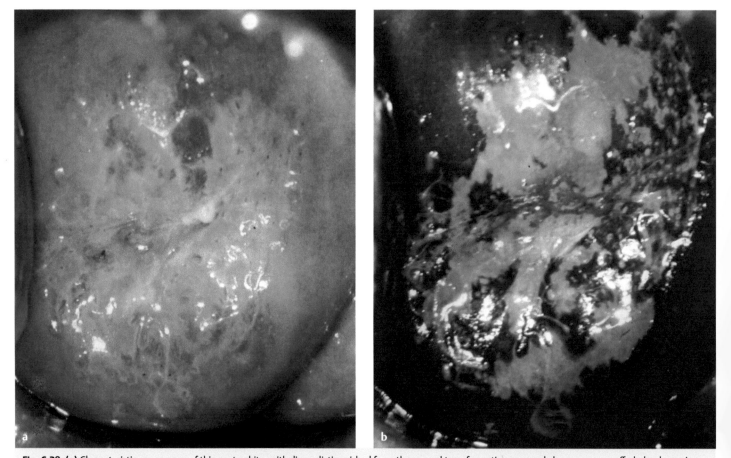

Fig. 6.28 **(a)** Characteristic appearance of thin acetowhite epithelium, distinguished from the normal transformation zone only by numerous cuffed gland openings. Histology showed low-grade squamous intraepithelial lesion (LSIL) (CIN 1). **(b)** Application of iodine (Schiller's test) reveals a variegated appearance resulting from the admixture of LSIL and fully mature brown squamous epithelium.

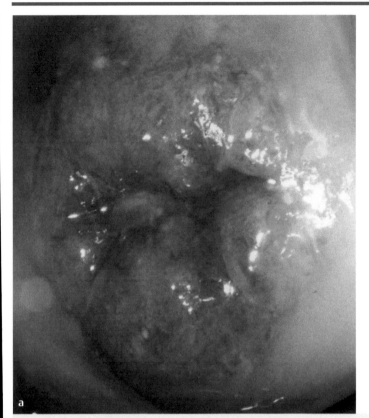
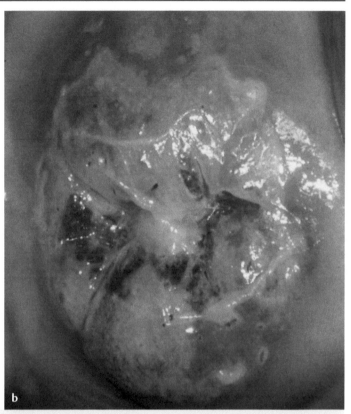

Fig. 6.29 (a) Before application of acetic acid, the white epithelium shows indistinct red tones. Several nabothian follicles shine through the reddish surface. **(b)** The white change is produced by acetic acid. Some gland openings are cuffed. The lesion between the 11 o'clock and 12 o'clock positions is due to glandular involvement. Histology showed LSIL (CIN 1).

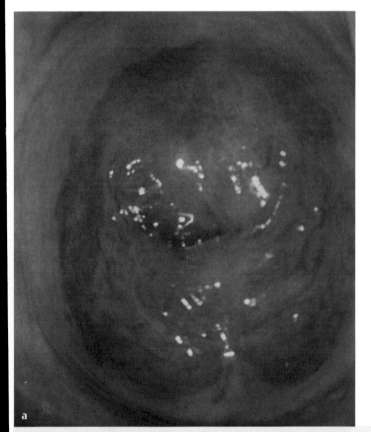
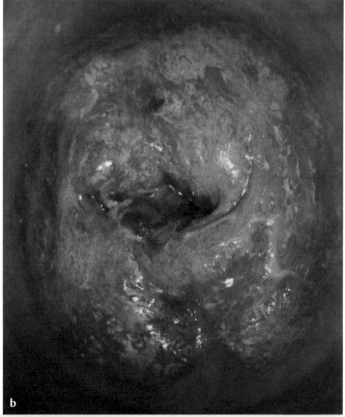

Fig. 6.30 (a) Pronounced red transformation zone, sharply demarcated from the original squamous epithelium. **(b)** Patchy appearance after application of acetic acid. Between the coarse and irregular white patches, there are reddish areas with cuffed gland openings and solid epithelial pegs in the glands. Histology showed HSIL (CIN 3).

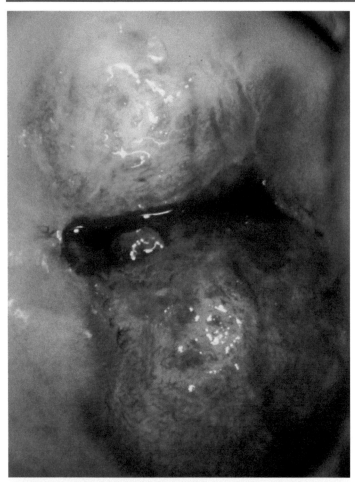

Fig. 6.31 Transformation zone with suspicious vessels on the posterior lip. Histology showed HSIL (CIN 3).

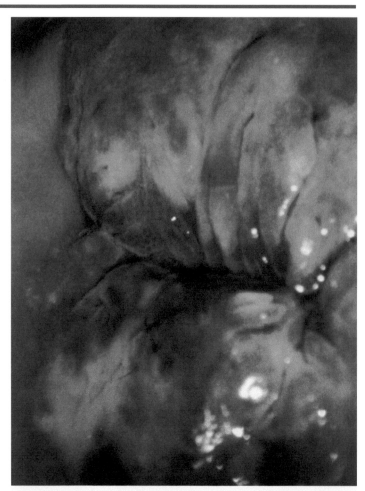

Fig. 6.32 Dense acetowhite epithelium after application of acetic acid. There are only isolated gland openings. Histology showed HSIL (CIN 3).

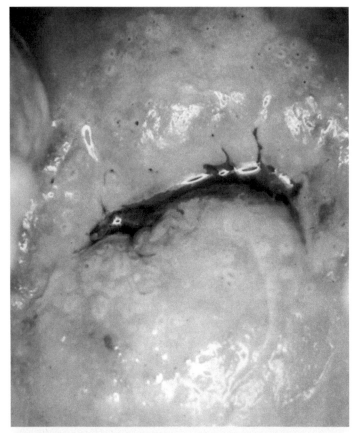

Fig. 6.33 Dense acetowhite epithelium with numerous cuffed gland openings. Histology showed HSIL (CIN 3).

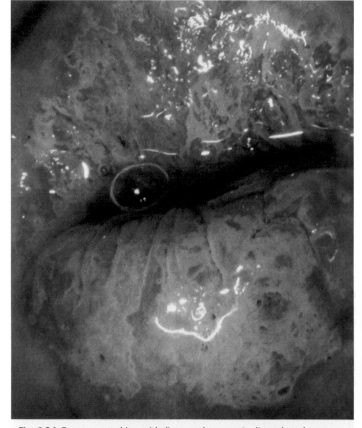

Fig. 6.34 Dense acetowhite epithelium on the posterior lip and on the anterior lip between 12 o'clock and 3 o'clock and between 9 o'clock and 10 o'clock positions. Histologically, the acetowhite epithelium was HSIL (CIN 3), whereas the pale pink area on the anterior lip was metaplastic epithelium.

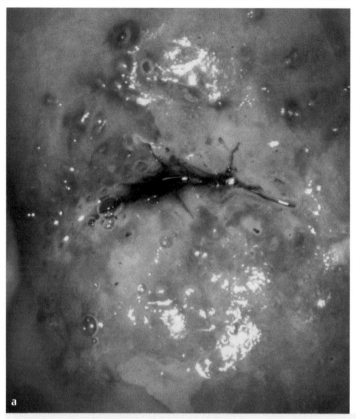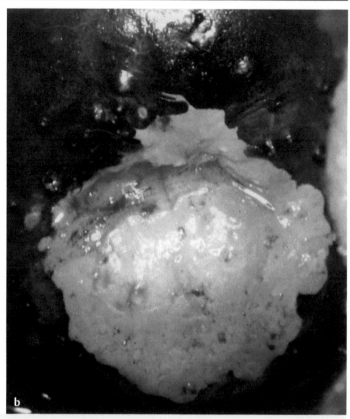

Fig. 6.35 **(a)** Dense acetowhite epithelium involving the entire posterior lip as well as the external os between 11 o'clock and 1 o'clock positions. Note the whiteness of the epithelium and the gland openings, some of which are cuffed. Histology showed HSIL (CIN 3). **(b)** After iodine staining, the pathologic epithelium clearly stands out against the fully mature squamous epithelium in the transformation zone.

6.2.2 Atypical Transformation Zone

The term *atypical transformation zone* was previously used as an umbrella designation for practically all abnormal colposcopic appearances such as leukoplakia, punctation, and mosaic, as these also occur outside the TZ. The term is no longer part of the official nomenclature.

6.2.3 Mosaic

The term *mosaic* refers to a colposcopic pattern of cobblestone-like tiles with capillaries forming the borders of the individual tiles. As with punctation, the appearances of mosaic are determined by epithelial changes, which allow distinction between *fine mosaic* (minor change) and *coarse mosaic* (major change).

Fine Mosaic

Fine mosaic, like fine punctation, occurs in sharply demarcated areas in the plane of the superficial epithelium. The appearance of such an area before application of acetic acid can be nonspecific and can remind one of a relatively vascular TZ, which, however, is usually devoid of gland openings or cysts (Figs. 6.27 and 6.36–6.42). A distinct color change to gray-white occurs with acetic acid application, and the margins become sharp. The blood vessels become less conspicuous (Fig. 6.27b). The whole area remains in the same plane as before. The mosaic pattern is delineated by the fine network of pale red lines. Such an area may not display the mosaic pattern throughout its entirety; in places, the surface may be uniform and flat because the epithelium is not supported by elongated stromal papillae.

It can be difficult to classify mosaic as fine or coarse (Figs. 6.39 and 6.42). Intermediate forms are mostly caused by low-grade

squamous intraepithelial lesion (LSIL), which may also produce various forms of punctation, depending on the degree of atypia and epithelial architecture.

Coarse Mosaic

Coarse mosaic is characterized by greater irregularity of the mosaic pattern. The network of fissures is more pronounced and intensely red. The furrows are more widely spaced, and the epithelial cobbles between them are bigger and more variable in shape than in the fine form (Figs. 6.38–6.41). The swelling from acetic acid makes the structures stand out (Fig. 6.41); the peak effect may take a minute to develop. The metamorphosis can be observed through the colposcope as the coarse structure of the mosaic and punctation gradually appears. In contrast, the effect of acetic acid on fine mosaic is immediate.

Gland openings and nabothian follicles are usually not found within areas of punctation or mosaic. Like leukoplakia, mosaic and punctation can also be found outside the TZ, in original squamous epithelium (Figs. 6.39, 6.43, and 6.44; see also Fig. 6.52). This is fundamental to the understanding of the morphogenesis of punctation and mosaic and epithelial atypia.

Punctation and mosaic occur in isolated fields (Figs. 6.39 and 6.43–6.45) and can coexist with other lesions (see Fig. 6.42; also see Fig. 7.20). In the latter case, the more peripherally located lesions usually represent lower-grade lesions (LSIL, CIN 1) or merely metaplastic epithelium, which was confirmed by topographic studies showing that mosaic and punctation occur more commonly outside than inside the TZ (84 vs. 16%). Histologically, mosaic and punctation outside the TZ corresponded to benign metaplastic epithelium in 70% and to CIN in only 30% of treated cases; within the TZ, the respective rates were 20 and 80%. Thus, mosaic and punctation within the TZ are more likely to represent CIN than are the same lesions outside the TZ.

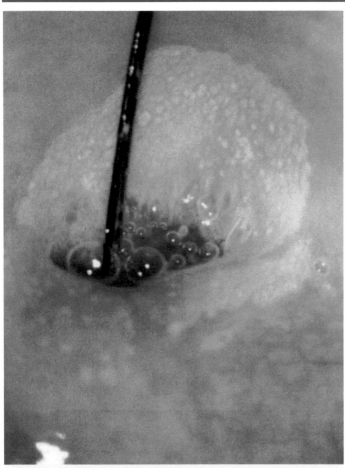

Fig. 6.36 Fine mosaic, mainly on the anterior lip of the external os, after application of acetic acid. Histology showed metaplastic epithelium. The string of an intrauterine device is visible.

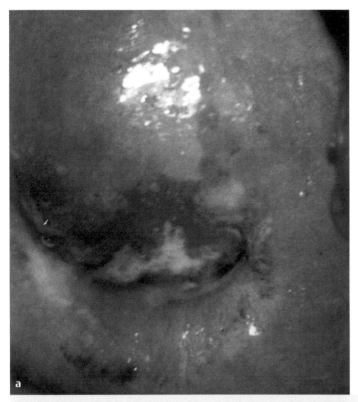

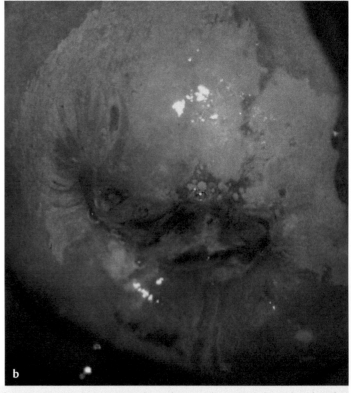

Fig. 6.37 (a) Indistinct lesion outside an intensely red area around the external os. Close examination shows increased vascularity on the posterior lip at the edge of the area. **(b)** Application of acetic acid shows an unexpectedly large, fine mosaic, mainly on the anterior lip. The whitish points in the narrow transformation zone are glands filled by squamous epithelium. Histology showed metaplastic epithelium.

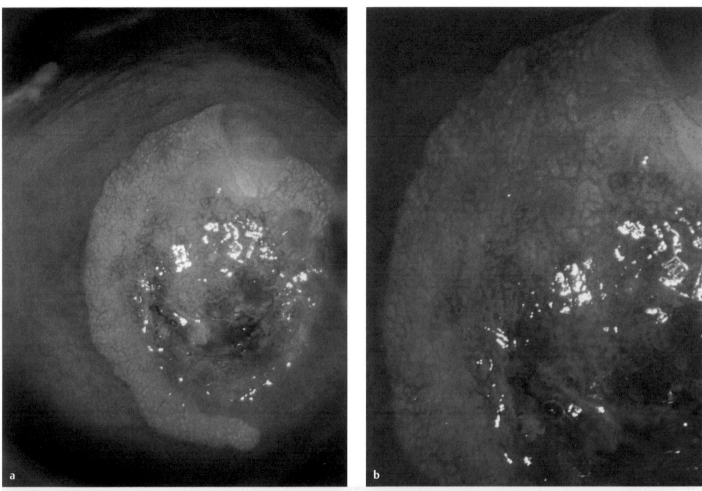

Fig. 6.38 **(a)** Transformation zone surrounded by a semicircular area that turns whitish after the application of acetic acid and shows a fine mosaic. **(b)** Higher magnification shows that the mosaic is coarser and more irregular than in Figs. 6.27, 6.36, and 6.37. Histology showed LSIL (CIN 1).

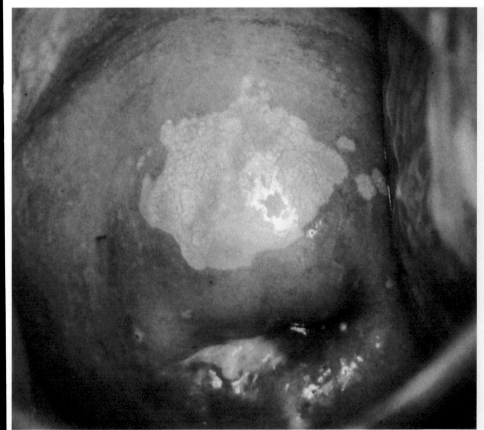

Fig. 6.39 Fine to coarse mosaic outside the transformation zone involving original squamous epithelium. Histology showed HSIL (CIN 2).

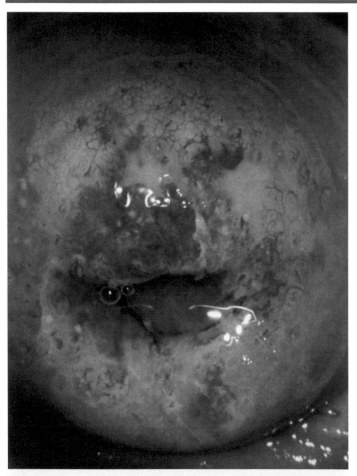

Fig. 6.40 Coarse mosaic around the os. Histology showed HSIL (CIN 3).

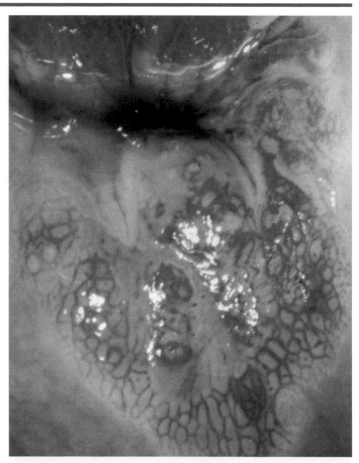

Fig. 6.41 Coarse mosaic intermingling with coarse punctation on the posterior lip. The border to the acetowhite epithelium is sharp, corresponding to HSIL (CIN 3). The mosaic returned HSIL (CIN 2).

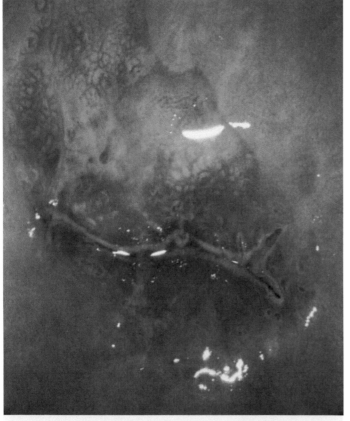

Fig. 6.42 Fine to coarse mosaic intermingling with fine punctation at the edge of acetowhite epithelium with cuffed gland openings and solid white points. The points correspond to HSIL (CIN 3).

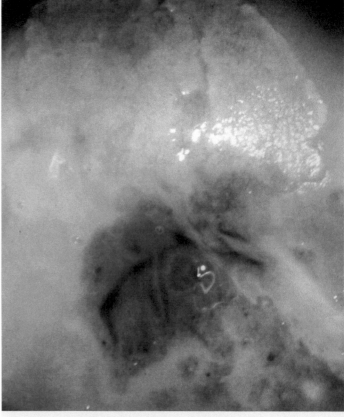

Fig. 6.43 Leukoplakia outside the transformation zone, on the anterior lip of the cervix. Histology showed metaplastic epithelium.

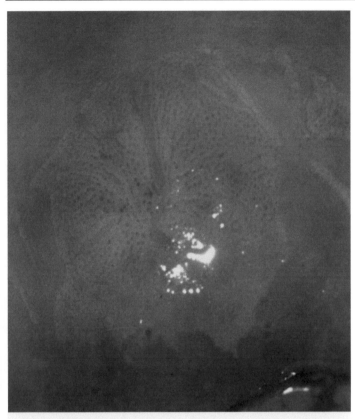

Fig. 6.44 Slightly prominent punctation. The entire sharply demarcated area apparently lies within unaltered squamous epithelium. Histology showed HSIL (CIN 3).

6.2.4 Punctation

Punctation is a colposcopic finding caused by capillary loops near to and visible through the epithelial surface as dots in a stippled pattern. Usually, punctation is imprinted on a uniform surface that is undisturbed by either gland openings or nabothian follicles or by any other signs of a TZ. The degree of punctation depends on the type of underlying epithelial abnormality. The type of punctation, as well as of mosaic, is important at colposcopic evaluation. The colposcopist should be aware that similar colposcopic appearances can be due to either benign metaplastic epithelium or atypical epithelium, which differ only in arrangement and degree of expression.

Two types of punctation are of diagnostic importance: *fine punctation* (minor change) and *coarse punctation* (major change). There are good diagnostic criteria to distinguish between the two types, but it is not always possible to categorize a given case as one or the other. Such appearances should always be regarded with suspicion: biopsy should be carried out, or cytology should be repeated.

Fine Punctation

Fine punctation characteristically imparts delicate stippling to an otherwise circumscribed grayish white to reddish area (Fig. 6.45). When the epithelium is keratinized, the dots may appear white, but they are usually red and remain in the same plane as the surface epithelium, even after the application of acetic acid. The "dots" of fine punctation are close together (Fig. 6.46). Fine punctation is often combined with equally fine mosaic. Fine focal punctation may be due to inflammation, in which case the

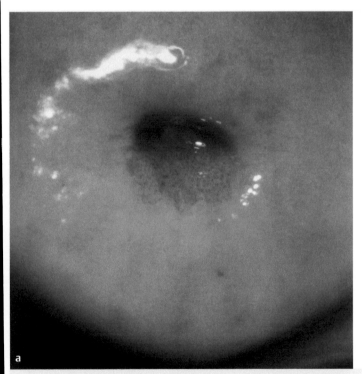

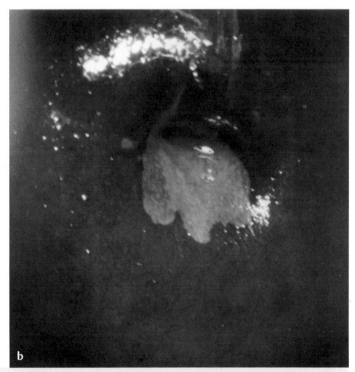

Fig. 6.45 (a) A fine punctation on the posterior lip of the cervix extends into the cervical canal. The squamocolumnar junction is not visible (type 3). (b) After application of iodine, the epithelium is stained brown. This so-called iodine-positive punctation is a sign of human papillomavirus infection. Histology showed LSIL (CIN 1) with koilocytosis.

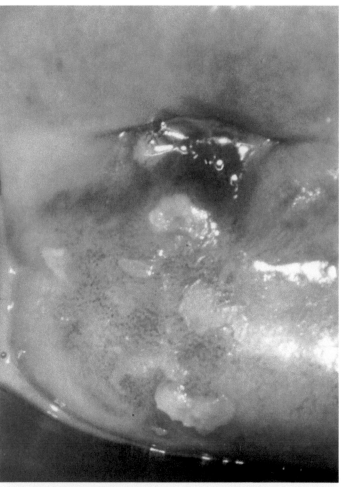

Fig. 6.46 Leukoplakia. Punctation appears where the keratin layer has been peeled off. Histology showed keratinizing metaplastic epithelium.

margins of the inflamed area appear indistinct after application of iodine (see Figs. 6.47 and 6.48b). Fine punctation can also be associated with LSIL (caused by human papillomavirus [HPV] infection). With the Schiller's iodine test, the punctations become yellow to ocher, whereas the adjacent epithelium, as a result of the koilocytes, stains brown. This is known as iodine-positive punctation (Fig. 6.45b).

Coarse Punctation

Coarse punctation usually indicates HSIL. The petechiae are more pronounced, bigger, and widely separated (Figs. 6.44 and 6.49–6.51). In extreme cases, punctation resembles papillae (Fig. 6.52). With higher magnification, corkscrew capillaries can be seen in the papillae. After application of acetic acid, coarse punctation stands out from the plane of the surrounding surface epithelium (Fig. 6.49a, b). Coarse punctation may be combined with coarse mosaic. The two patterns may overlap, with intermingling of dots and fissures (Fig. 6.50).

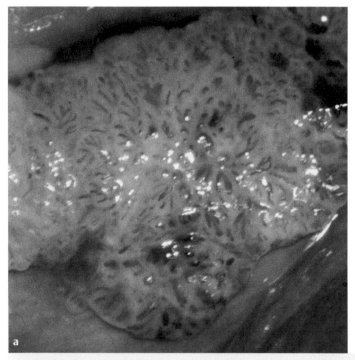

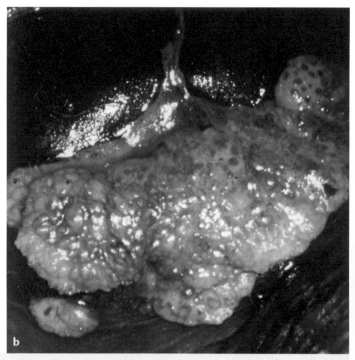

Fig. 6.47 **(a)** On higher magnification, the vessels within the papillae resemble commas and antlers. Their coarseness gives the impression of atypia. **(b)** Condyloma. The brownish color after application of iodine indicates glycogen-containing patches within the condyloma and correlates well with the histologic picture.

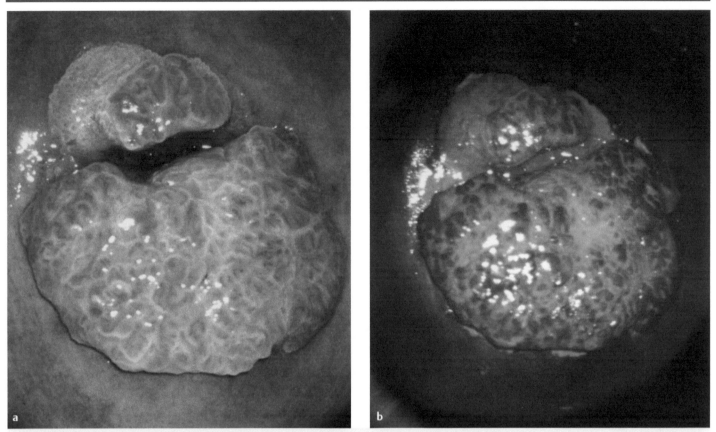

Fig. 6.48 **(a)** Exophytic condylomatous lesion after application of 3% acetic acid. **(b)** After application of iodine, the surface shows the patchy brown staining typical of condylomas and an ocher epithelium.

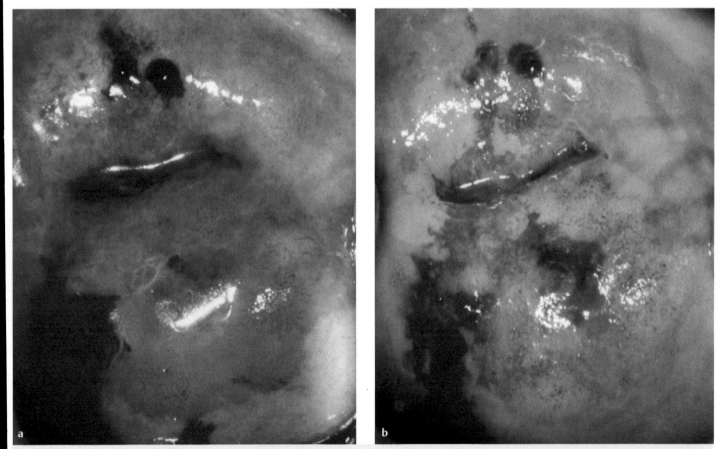

Fig. 6.49 **(a)** Atypical yellowish-reddish area showing focal coarse punctation. **(b)** After application of acetic acid, the area of punctation swells, stands out from the surface, and becomes white. Histology showed HSIL (CIN 3). There is an island of fully mature squamous epithelium in the transformation zone on the anterior lip.

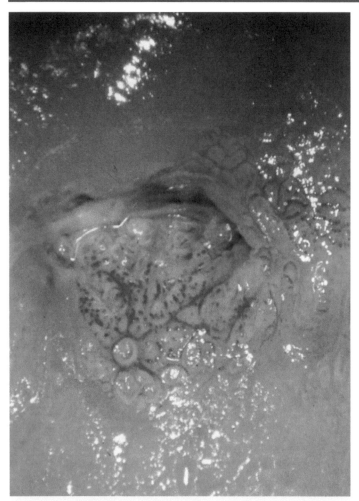

Fig. 6.50 Combination of coarse punctation and coarse mosaic. Histology showed HSIL (CIN 3).

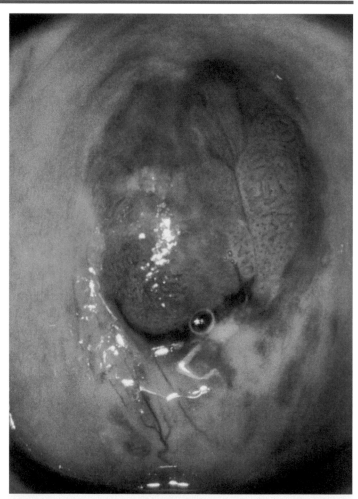

Fig. 6.51 Coarse, irregular punctation before the application of acetic acid. Histology showed HSIL (CIN 2). On the posterior lip, there is a regular vascular pattern in a mature transformation zone.

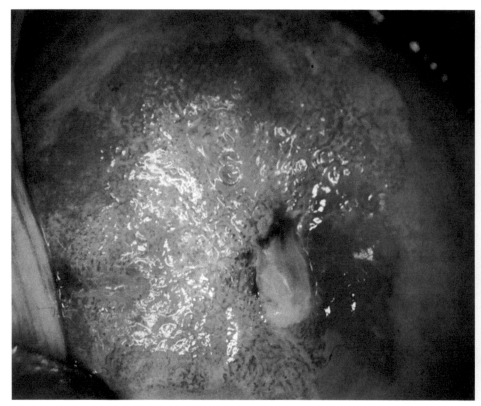

Fig. 6.52 Coarse punctation. Note the papillary appearance. Histology showed HSIL with early stromal invasion (FIGO stage IA1).

6.2.5 Leukoplakia (Keratosis)

Leukoplakia (keratosis) can usually be seen with the naked eye (Figs. 6.53 and 6.54a, b), but sometimes the colposcope is necessary (Fig. 6.55). Histologically, leukoplakia corresponds to parakeratosis or true keratinization, which cannot be distinguished colposcopically. A colposcopically delicate white patch, however, usually corresponds to parakeratosis, whereas hyperkeratosis usually produces a thick, rough-surfaced plaque. Fine leukoplakias are well circumscribed (Fig. 6.55), their surface either flat or finely pitted. When keratinization is marked, the margins become obscured by the overlapping horny layer. The surface may be smooth but is more commonly pitted and may even have a mosaic appearance. Partial shedding or removal of the keratin can result in a plaque-like appearance, referred to as *plaque-like* or *thick leukoplakia*.

If the keratin layer is completely wiped away, the underlying epithelium can display a pattern, often punctation (Fig. 6.46). Leukoplakia can be found within or outside the TZ, in the latter case arising from original squamous epithelium.

It is important to appreciate that the type of epithelium underlying leukoplakia cannot be predicted colposcopically. The epithelium may be of metaplastic origin, especially when the leukoplakia is fine. When cornification is more pronounced, the underlying epithelium may show the features of HSIL (CIN 3), early stromal invasion (ESI) (Fig. 6.54), even deeper invasion, or only benign acanthosis (Fig. 6.43). Even iodine staining (Schiller's test) cannot provide further diagnostic clues (Fig. 6.54b). Moderate-sized leukoplakias typically stain canary yellow with iodine, which also enhances their sharp demarcation.

Leukoplakias usually should be evaluated with biopsy. Neither the surface contour nor the location of leukoplakia with regard to the TZ can predict whether the underlying epithelium is benign or neoplastic. Cytology is not diagnostic because the smear contains largely cornified material and nothing representative from an underlying lesion. Topographic studies have shown that leukoplakia is usually found outside the TZ and that it corresponds histologically to benign metaplastic epithelium in 62% of cases and to SIL in 38%.

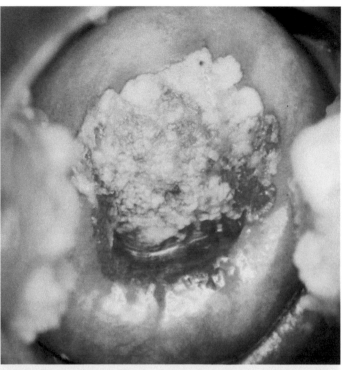

Fig. 6.53 Coarse plaque of keratosis with a partly fissured surface. Histology showed HSIL (CIN 3).

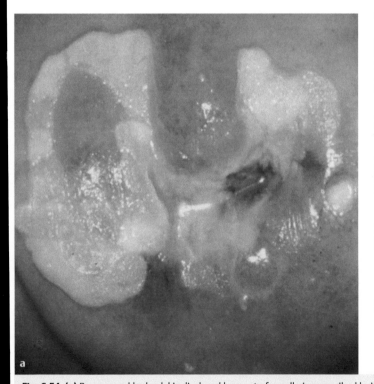

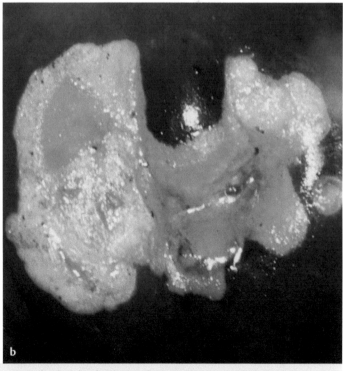

Fig. 6.54 (a) Pronounced leukoplakia displayed by most of a well-circumscribed lesion. Note the sharp border close to the external os at 11 o'clock position. Conization showed HSIL with early stromal invasion (FIGO stage IA1). **(b)** After application of iodine, the border seen in **(a)** is accentuated. The leukoplakia is outside the transformation zone. A plaque-like arrangement of the keratin is suggested.

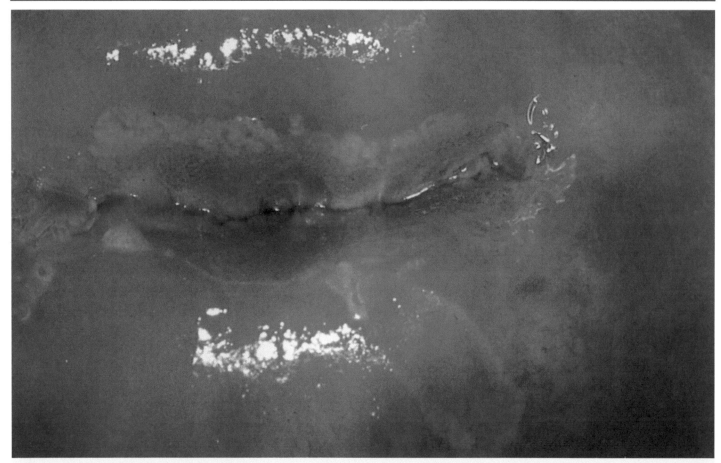

Fig. 6.55 Sharply demarcated but only slightly keratotic area on the posterior lip of the cervix. Histology showed metaplastic epithelium with parakeratosis. Note the thin seam of transformation zone on the anterior lip.

6.2.6 Erosion and Ulcer

Erosions are superficial epithelial defects; deeper defects, with exposure of the stroma, are called *ulcers*. Erosions and ulcerations are not normal during the reproductive years but can be iatrogenic artifacts during examination in the atrophic postmenopausal epithelium, particularly when obtaining the smear. Atypical epithelium is particularly vulnerable as it lacks cohesiveness, being more loosely structured than normal squamous epithelium. This accounts for the exfoliation of cells detected in smears as well as the swelling induced by acetic acid. The epithelium is also less firmly attached to the underlying stroma, from which it may detach easily to produce an erosion.

Ulcers are less easy to see when they occur within a colposcopically evident lesion (Fig. 6.56). They are seen better with iodine because the exposed stroma does not stain (Fig. 6.55b). An ulcer can be recognized by its intense red color, granular floor, and punched-out margin (Figs. 6.57 and 6.58). It is important not to miss larger ulcers that result from detachment of whole epithelial fields (Fig. 6.58). Careful examination of the edges of such defects will reveal residual epithelium, which differs from surrounding normal epithelium in its color and acetic acid reaction. Biopsy should be performed on such epithelial rims.

Endophytic carcinomas (Fig. 6.59) can masquerade as erosions or flat ulcers, so flat ulcers should be probed with a Chrobak's sound (Fig. 3.4). Stroma infiltrated by tumor offers no resistance; the sound advances as into warm butter. With normal tissues, the probe encounters firm elastic resistance.

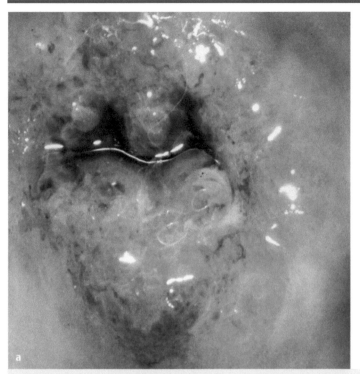
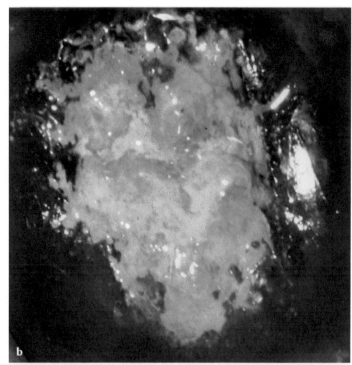

Fig. 6.56 **(a)** True erosion at the outskirts of an acetowhite epithelium. The step-like edge, with pathologic as well as normal squamous epithelium, is well shown in places. Biopsy of the whitish epithelium showed HSIL (CIN 2). **(b)** After application of iodine, the pathologic epithelium is typically iodine-yellow, whereas the erosion does not stain at all.

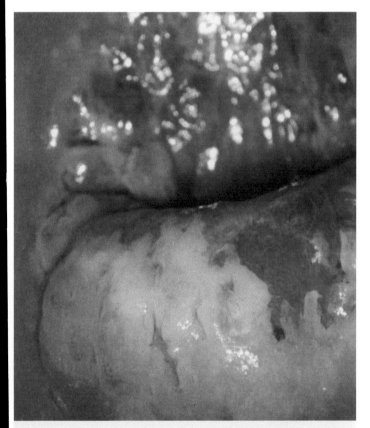

Fig. 6.57 Typical erosion in white epithelium. Epithelial denudation reveals the intensely red stroma. Histology of the whitish epithelium showed HSIL (CIN 3).

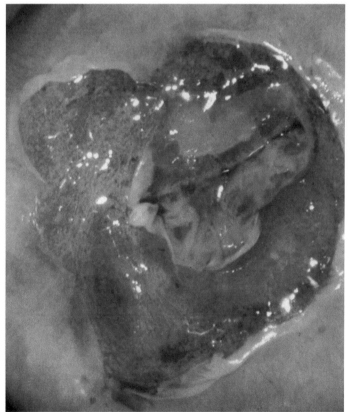

Fig. 6.58 Extensive erosion. Islands of HSIL (CIN 3) remain both toward the endocervical canal and bordering the peripheral, normal squamous epithelium. The texture of the stroma is exposed.

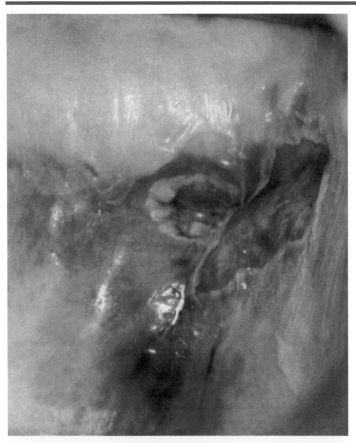

Fig. 6.59 Flat ulcer to the left of the external os. Its floor is uneven and yellowish to dark red. Histology showed squamous cell carcinoma (FIGO stage IB).

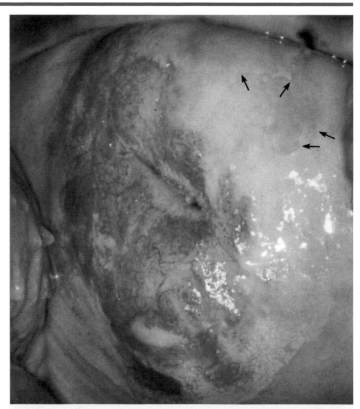

Fig. 6.60 Markedly vascular transformation zone. At the periphery, between 4 o'clock and 6 o'clock positions, there is a moderately coarse mosaic as well as clearly delineated mild keratosis. Conization and histology showed early stromal invasion (FIGO stage IA1) of a squamous lesion and metaplastic epithelium at the white plaques.

6.2.7 Signs of Early Invasive Carcinoma

Colposcopic detection of small invasive lesions depends on how big and where the lesions are. Foci of ESI, which reach only a fraction of a millimeter into the cervical stroma, cannot be seen with the colposcope. Also, such foci arise more often from glands involved by SIL than from atypical surface epithelium. In the latter case, the colposcopic appearance is that of the parent epithelium.

The colposcopic signs of ESI are indirect. The likelihood of ESI increases with the surface extent of a lesion. Also, ESI is more common when simultaneously there are different types of epithelia. Some cases show all these features. Increased vascularity also suggests invasion (Figs. 6.60 and 6.61).

Although the likelihood of ESI increases with the size of a lesion, quite small or poorly vascularized lesions can be invasive. Some cases of ESI have surprisingly few colposcopic changes (Figs. 6.62–6.64).

Similarly, colposcopic detection of *microinvasive carcinomas* depends on their size and location. If a microinvasive carcinoma is entirely within the cervical canal, the ectocervix will show no clue. Ectocervical lesions characterized by focal collections of atypical vessels are highly suspicious for microinvasion. Atypical vessels are invariably restricted to the invasive focus (Figs. 6.65–6.68). The vessels are often drawn out, have an irregular course, and are prone to bleed.

Somewhat larger cervical cancers can produce a slight bump on the surface that gives away their location (Figs. 6.66 and 6.67), or they can form a confined polypoid lesion (Fig. 6.69a, b). The diagnosis of an invasive lesion arising within an already vascular TZ is difficult, if not impossible. Hints of invasion in such cases may be sought only retrospectively by carefully correlating the colposcopic findings with the histology of the conization specimen (Fig. 6.68).

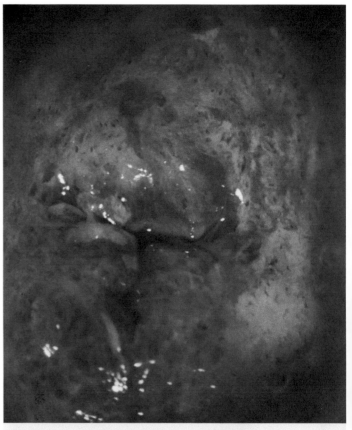

Fig. 6.61 Dense acetowhite epithelium with a strikingly coarse surface. There are irregularly located, comma-shaped vessels in the entire area. The conization specimen showed HSIL (CIN 2/3) and early stromal invasion (FIGO stage IA1).

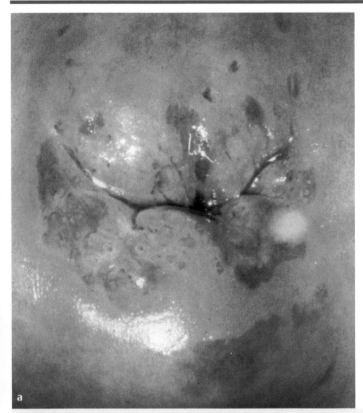 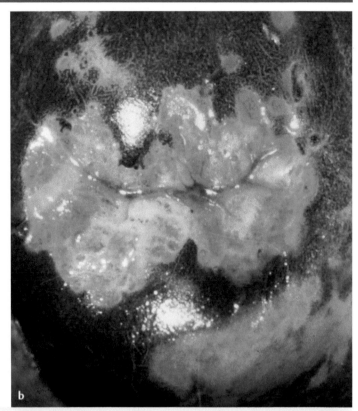

Fig. 6.62 (a) Acetowhite epithelium that merges imperceptibly with the periphery. Note the separate poorly circumscribed reddish area on the posterior lip. **(b)** The iodine-yellow area around the external os was HSIL (CIN 3) with early stromal invasion (FIGO stage IA1). The isolated area on the posterior lip was inflammatory. The speckled brown lesion on the anterior lip is condylomatous colpitis (Fig. 6.103).

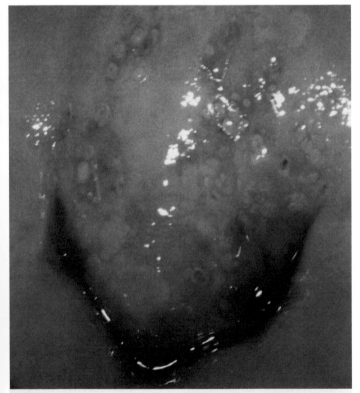 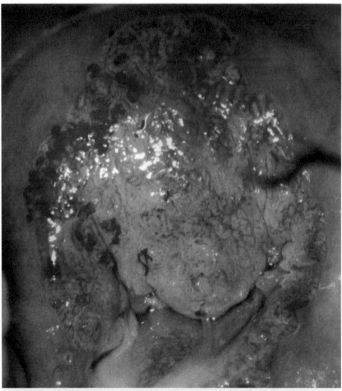

Fig. 6.63 Acetowhite epithelium with cuffed gland openings after application of acetic acid. The conization specimen showed HSIL (CIN 3) with early stromal invasion (FIGO stage IA1).

Fig. 6.64 Acetowhite epithelium and coarse mosaic after application of 3% acetic acid. Note the friability of the extensive lesion. Histology showed HSIL (CIN 3) with early stromal invasion (FIGO stage IA1).

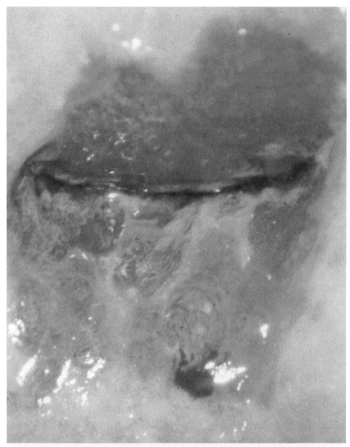

Fig. 6.65 White epithelium before acetic acid application harboring a FIGO stage IA2 microinvasive squamous cell carcinoma just above the bleeding point. Note the irregularly branching vessels. The neighboring reddish areas corresponded to HSIL (CIN 3). True erosion and regenerating epithelium can be seen in the vicinity of the external os on the posterior lip and regenerating epithelium on the anterior lip.

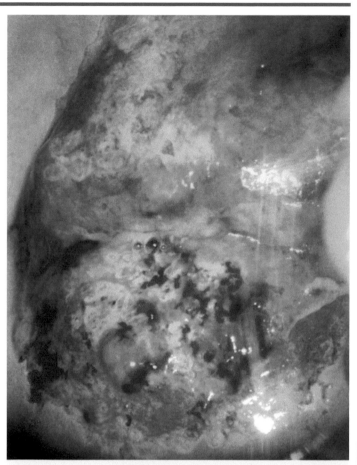

Fig. 6.66 Large area of white epithelium before application of acetic acid. The surface of the posterior lip is bulging because of the presence of a small FIGO stage IB1 carcinoma. Note the extravasation of blood where the vessels are atypical.

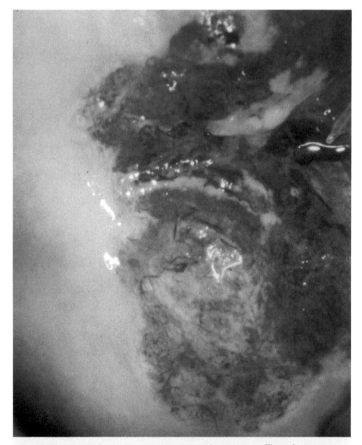

Fig. 6.67 Stage IA2 microinvasive carcinoma (squamous cell) producing a small bulge on the posterior lip. Atypical vessels course over the white surface.

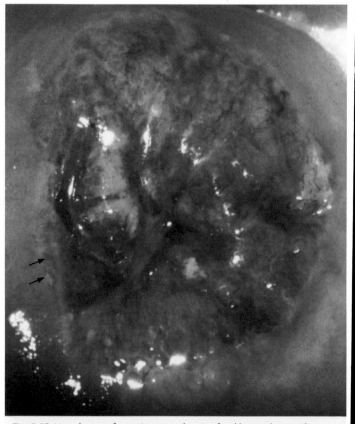

Fig. 6.68 Vascular transformation zone showing focal hemorrhages. The microinvasive carcinoma (FIGO stage IA2) occupying the left lateral recess of the external os is easily overlooked.

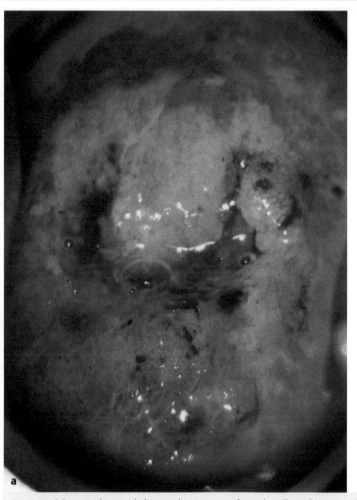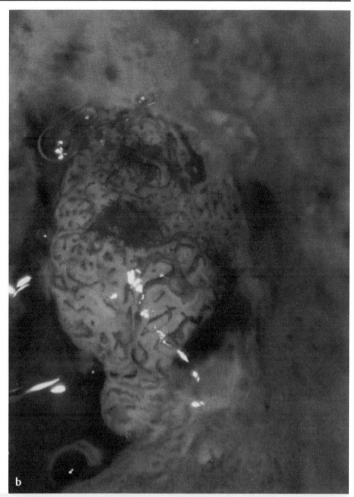

Fig. 6.69 (a) Acetowhite epithelium with a coarse surface. The effect of acetic acid is especially marked on the anterior lip: white epithelium with a small polypoid lesion in the left corner of the external os. **(b)** At high magnification, the tumor shows numerous atypical vessels. The polypoid structure is a small, exophytic stage IB1 carcinoma (squamous cell).

6.2.8 Invasive Carcinoma

Invasive carcinomas on the ectocervix can be seen with the naked eye. Tumors located entirely within the cervical canal can be seen better with the colposcope, but only if the os is somewhat gaping. In all other cases, colposcopy merely confirms the gross findings. The degree of distortion of the ectocervical contour depends on the growth pattern of the tumor. Exophytic lesions protrude into the vagina as fungating tumors of varying size (Figs. 6.70–6.72). In contrast, purely endophytic neoplasms present merely as red or white eroded areas, the true nature of which can be recognized only by their papillary surface and atypical vessels (Fig. 6.73). Flat endophytic carcinomas with ulcerated surfaces can be difficult to diagnose both with the naked eye and with the colposcope (Fig. 6.74). In such cases, palpation and probing with a Chrobak's sound (Fig. 3.4) are of value. Most invasive carcinomas are partly exophytic and partly endophytic, and their diagnosis should pose no difficulty. Most carcinomas surround the external os (Figs. 6.71 and 6.75). Less often, one or only part of one lip is involved (Figs. 6.76 and 6.77).

The surface of invasive tumors is usually irregularly fissured (Fig. 6.78) like a cauliflower. If the papillae are somewhat finer and more regular, they can be confused with ectopy. The degree of ulceration and tissue destruction is greater in more advanced cancers. Occasionally, tumors present as smooth sessile polyps (Fig. 6.77), to be distinguished from benign polyps by their vasculature and by use of Chrobak's sound (Fig. 3.4).

An endophytic tumor with a keratotic surface can pose a further diagnostic challenge (Fig. 6.79). Performing biopsies of keratotic lesions will avoid missing lesions hidden by keratin.

Invasive cancers afford an excellent opportunity to study all kinds of atypical vessels (Figs. 6.69 and 6.141). This should be done after the cervix is cleansed with a dry swab and before applying acetic acid, which makes the vessels blanch (Fig. 6.80a, b). Invasive lesions also become more prominent and whitish with acetic acid (Fig. 6.80). After acetic acid, the criteria for the evaluation of atypical epithelia can be applied to preinvasive lesions, which frequently surround an invasive tumor (Fig. 6.78).

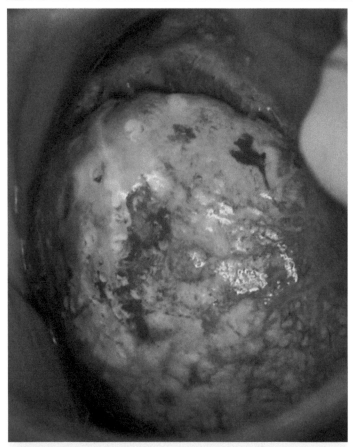

Fig. 6.70 Exophytic stage IB1 squamous cell carcinoma on the posterior lip. The tip is ulcerated.

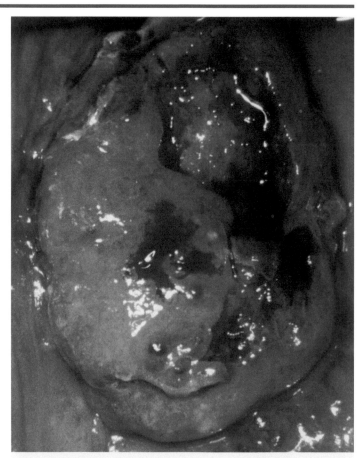

Fig. 6.71 Exophytic FIGO stage IB1 cervical carcinoma measuring 4 × 3 cm.

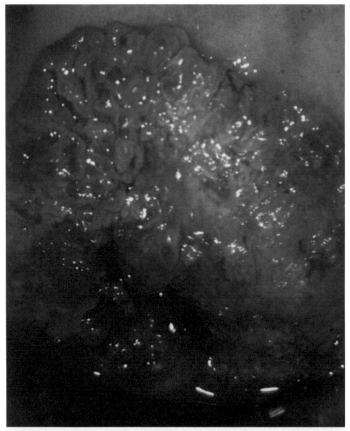

Fig. 6.72 Exophytic, papillary verrucous carcinoma around the external os (FIGO stage IB1).

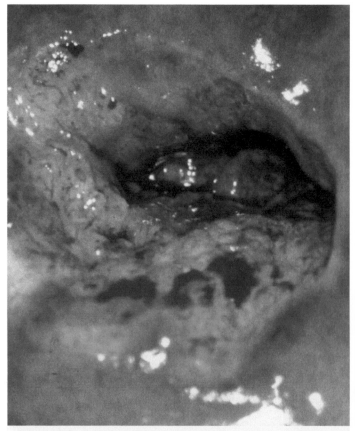

Fig. 6.73 FIGO stage IB1 squamous cell carcinoma after application of 3% acetic acid. The vessels are atypical and friable, and the surface is irregular.

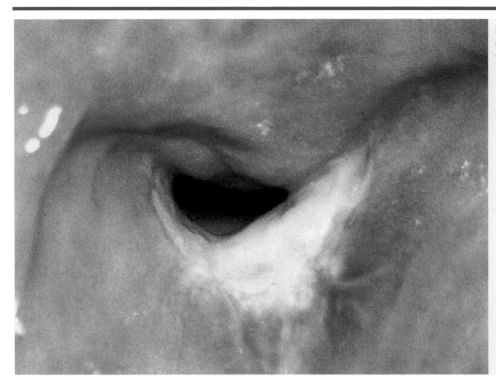

Fig. 6.74 Endophytic stage IB2 squamous carcinoma. Colposcopy shows a patulous external os and leukoplakia on the posterior lip of the cervix.

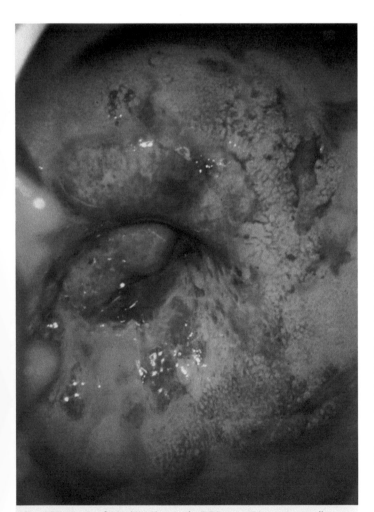

Fig. 6.75 Margin of HSIL (CIN 3) around a FIGO stage IB1 squamous cell carcinoma situated predominantly in the canal. Note the flat ulcer on the anterior lip surrounded by a coarse mosaic.

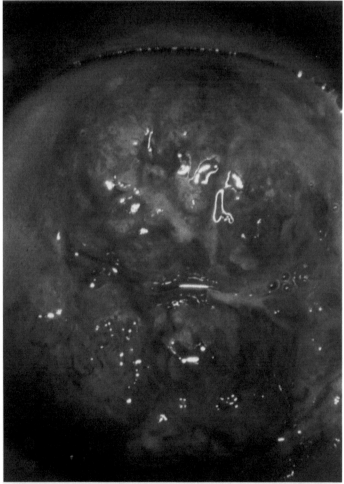

Fig. 6.76 This endophytic FIGO stage IB1 squamous cell carcinoma could be mistaken for white epithelium. The markedly atypical blood vessels on the posterior lip are associated invasive carcinomas.

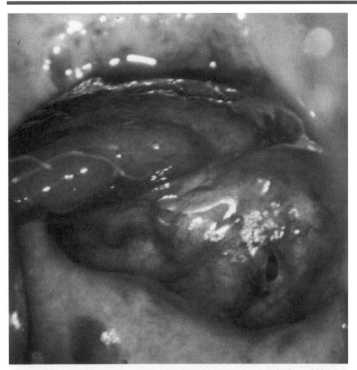

Fig. 6.77 Polypoid FIGO stage IB1 squamous cell carcinoma, which could be mistaken for a large benign cervical polyp. The color and blood supply of the polyp lower down resemble a nabothian follicle.

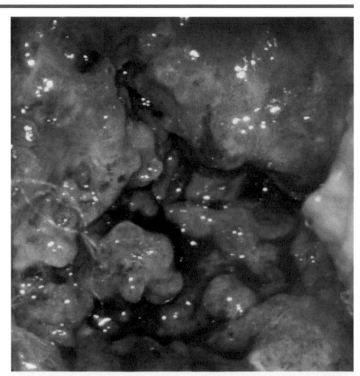

Fig. 6.78 Deeply fissured and coarsely papillary FIGO stage IIB squamous cell carcinoma. The vascular pattern is not pronounced.

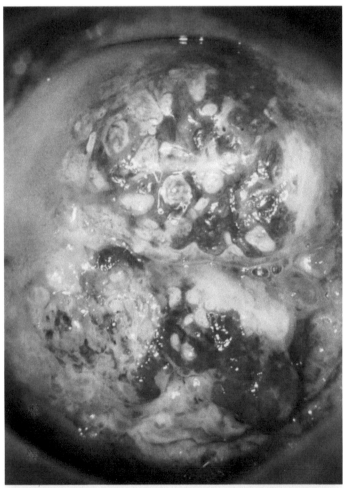

Fig. 6.79 Endophytic FIGO stage IB1 squamous cell carcinoma with marked hyperkeratosis.

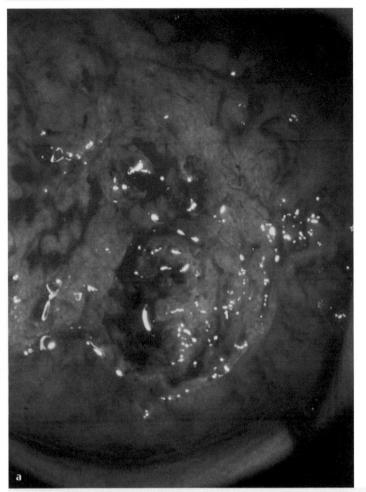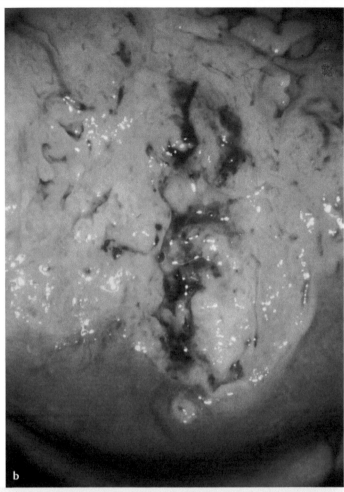

Fig. 6.80 **(a)** An exophytic FIGO stage IB1 squamous cell carcinoma with a variety of atypical blood vessels. **(b)** Application of acetic acid suppresses the vascular pattern and turns the background white.

6.2.9 Adenocarcinoma In Situ and Microinvasive Adenocarcinoma

There are no colposcopic images that are pathognomonic for the presence of an adenocarcinoma in situ (AIS) or a microinvasive adenocarcinoma. However, surface patterns indicative of AIS are lesions overlying columnar epithelium not contiguous with the squamocolumnar border, lesions with large gland openings, papillary lesions showing epithelial budding, and variegated red and white lesions. Because these lesions usually occur with SIL, one finds the colposcopic changes suggesting SIL (Figs. 6.81 and 6.82). Furthermore, AIS is usually located in glands or crypts; when on the surface, it is friable and often eroded (Figs. 6.81 and 6.83). The somewhat larger microinvasive adenocarcinoma can occasionally be seen with the colposcope but cannot reliably be distinguished from its squamous cell counterpart (Fig. 6.83).

6.3 Miscellaneous Colposcopic Findings

6.3.1 Nonsuspicious Iodine-Yellow Area

Regular use of the Schiller's (iodine) test frequently shows sharply circumscribed iodine-yellow areas that are otherwise either not visible or overlooked. Such areas are especially striking if the cervix at first sight appears completely normal (Fig. 6.84a). If the patient can be re-examined after the iodine reaction has

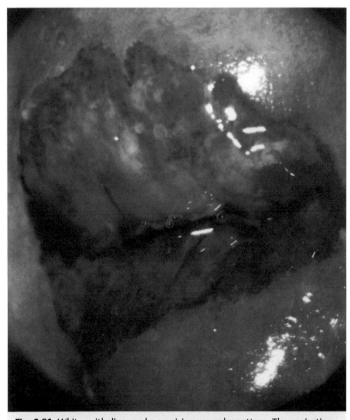

Fig. 6.81 White epithelium and a suspicious vascular pattern. The conization specimen showed LSIL (CIN 1) and HSIL (CIN 3) as well as an adenocarcinoma in situ (AIS) on the ectocervix. The latter was present both in glands and in the superficial columnar epithelium.

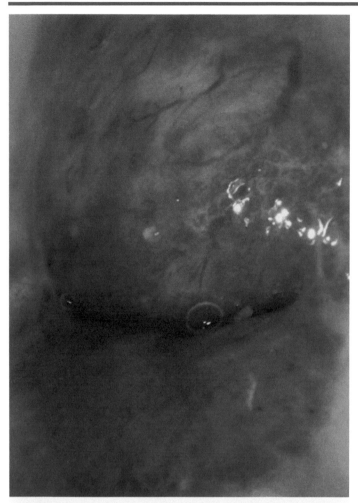

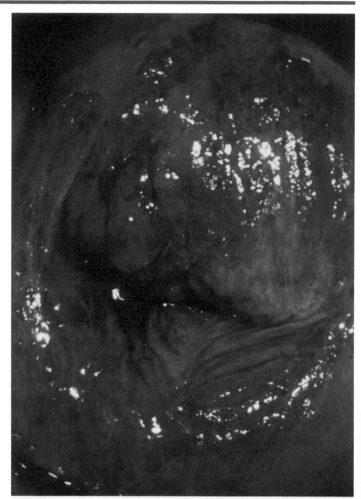

Fig. 6.82 White epithelium with a few gland openings. Histology showed HSIL (CIN 2) on the ectocervix and an adenocarcinoma in situ (AIS) in the lower part of the cervical canal.

Fig. 6.83 Large, partly eroded transformation zone. The rugae of the everted cervical mucosa are still visible. Histology of the whitish areas showed HSIL (CIN 2) and, on the left side of the cervical os, a 10 × 3-mm adenocarcinoma (FIGO stage IB1).

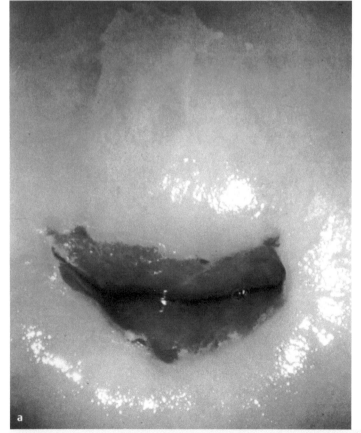

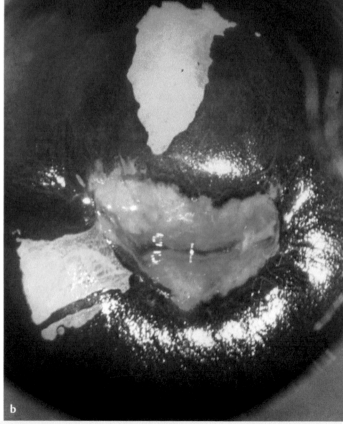

Fig. 6.84 **(a)** Only nuances in color suggest a lesion arising in original squamous epithelium. Such a lesion can be easily overlooked at routine colposcopy. **(b)** After application of iodine, the bright yellow area stands out. There is also a second yellow lesion, hardly recognizable in (a). Histology showed metaplastic epithelium.

abated, the previously iodine-yellow area will appear grayish and sharply demarcated.

Besides such unsuspected and isolated foci, iodine-yellow areas are also found in combination with other colposcopic lesions; the latter are therefore really bigger and have different outlines from first suspected (Fig. 6.85b).

Colposcopically nonsuspicious iodine-yellow areas are usually caused by benign metaplastic epithelium. The risk of intraepithelial neoplasia is low.

Transformation that has resulted in metaplastic squamous epithelium with colposcopic findings of a nonsuspect iodine-yellow area will not undergo further change (Fig. 6.86a–c).

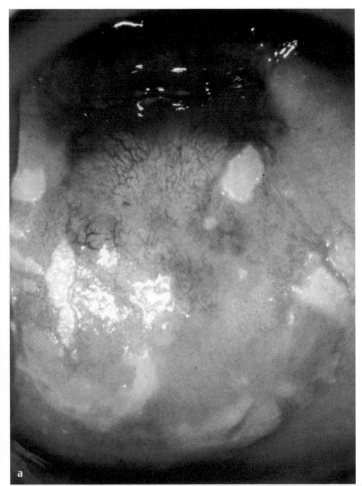 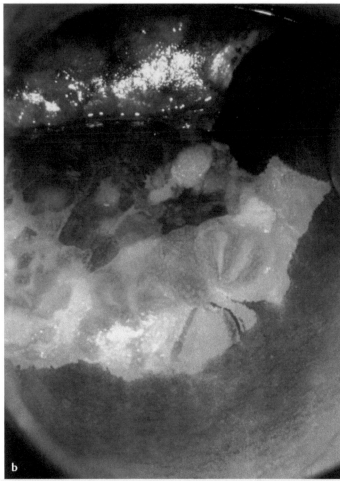

Fig. 6.85 (a) Keratoses in a vascular transformation zone. **(b)** The vascular epithelium stains strongly with iodine; the presence of the clearly circumscribed iodine-yellow areas was not suspected. Histology showed HSIL (CIN 3).

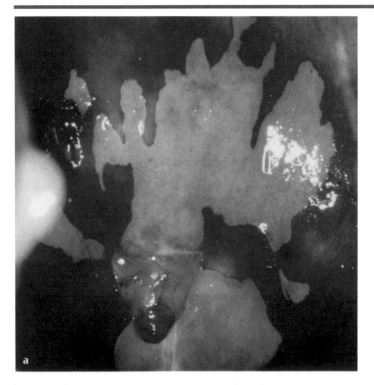

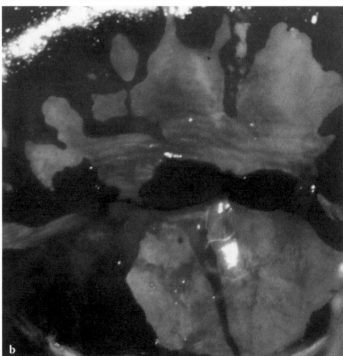

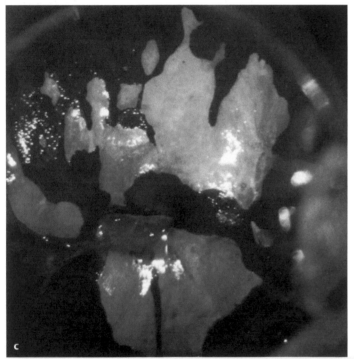

Fig. 6.86 (a–c) Bizarrely shaped nonsuspicious iodine-yellow areas. The contours remained unchanged over a 5-year period.

6.3.2 Congenital Transformation Zone

The congenital TZ is a colposcopic finding of a large iodine-yellow area extending into the anterior or posterior fornix (Fig. 6.87). This is a relatively common finding (4%), and the colposcopist should be thoroughly familiar with its appearance. The origin of this finding is unclear. It appears to be a variant of müllerian epithelial differentiation.

The epithelium is nonglycogenated and is faintly acetowhite; usually the degree of acetowhiteness is very minor and may be difficult to see. It can be recognized clearly after the application of Schiller's iodine. It has histologic features in common with squamous metaplasia.

A congenital TZ does not require biopsy or treatment.

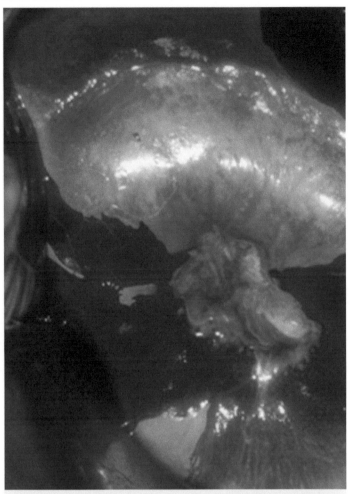

Fig. 6.87 Congenital transformation zone after the application of iodine.

6.3.3 Condylomatous Lesions

Colposcopy is important for the recognition of flat condylomatous lesions on the cervix. Such changes closely mimic suspicious findings but are benign and can be reversible. Condylomatous lesions (Figs. 6.47, 6.48, and 6.88–6.98) can coexist with SIL.

Condylomata acuminata are usually straightforward to diagnose colposcopically. However, an isolated condyloma in the region of the external os can be mistaken for an exophytic carcinoma (Fig. 6.88). Chrobak's probe can be a useful diagnostic aid (see Chapter 3). The surface of condylomatous lesions is classically papillary (Figs. 6.88–6.90, 6.94a, b, and 6.95). The structural details, however, can be concealed by keratin, resulting in a smooth, shiny, mother-of-pearl–like surface (Figs. 6.91 and 6.92). Not uncommonly, the papillae are fine and finger-like (Fig. 6.96). The color of condylomas varies according to the degree of keratinization and ranges from white and grayish red to intense red.

Condylomas are often multiple (Figs. 6.88 and 6.94) and vary in size, providing a good opportunity to study their development. Exophytic condylomas can intermingle with flat lesions (Fig. 6.94). Higher magnification reveals the presence of blood vessels within the papillae of condylomas. The vessels can be comma, corkscrew, or staghorn in shape and can appear suspicious because of their relatively large caliber (Fig. 6.47a, b). Flat and smooth lesions tend to have a distinctive pearly surface as a result of hyperkeratosis (Figs. 6.92 and 6.94). No criteria have been described to distinguish colposcopically between typical and atypical condylomas. However, the latter may have a coarser structure producing coarse punctation or mosaic by analogy with SIL (CIN) and metaplastic epithelium.

Application of iodine (Schiller's test) shows that condylomatous cells still contain some glycogen. A stippled, variegated appearance can be produced by focal keratinization (Figs. 6.93b, 6.47b, and 6.48a, b). Occasionally, glycogen storage by condylomatous epithelium produces the unusual colposcopic appearance of *iodine-positive mosaic or punctation* (Fig. 6.97a, b). It is unclear whether this picture is typical of condylomas, but at any rate, such mosaics are caused by glycogen-containing epithelium associated with tall stromal papillae. Histologically, the epithelium in such cases shows features suggestive of flat condylomas. An iodine-positive mosaic pattern can be produced by colposcopic lesions that, before the Schiller's test, appear nonspecific apart from their pearly surface. The result of the Schiller's test in such cases is all the more surprising (Fig. 6.98a, b).

Experienced colposcopists will have come across an essentially normal cervix and vagina, the surfaces of which are evenly studded with numerous white dots (Figs. 6.99 and 6.100). These correspond to the tips of elongated stromal papillae that perforate a rather irregular-structured yet glycogen-containing epithelium and is due to HPV infection. Meisels et al called this *condylomatous vaginitis*.

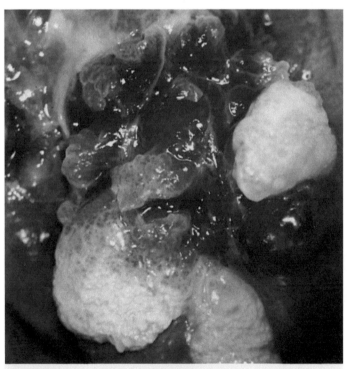

Fig. 6.88 Multiple condylomas around the external os. Only the tips of the large condylomas show advanced keratinization.

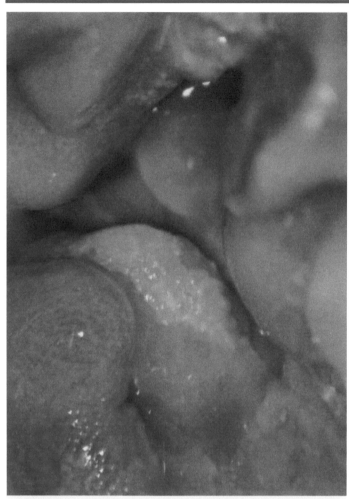

Fig. 6.89 Lacerated external os. Note the slightly elevated, fine papillary condyloma in a crease, not easily visible to the naked eye.

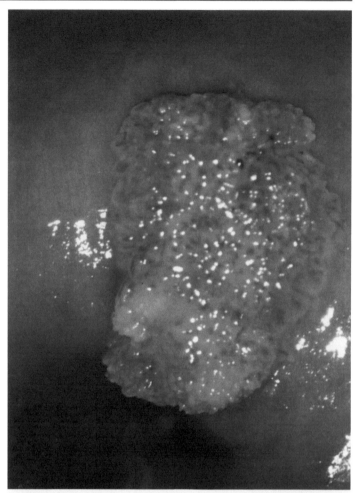

Fig. 6.90 Fine papillary, HPV 16—positive condyloma as an isolated lesion on the anterior lip of the cervix close to the external os. Histology showed a condyloma without atypia.

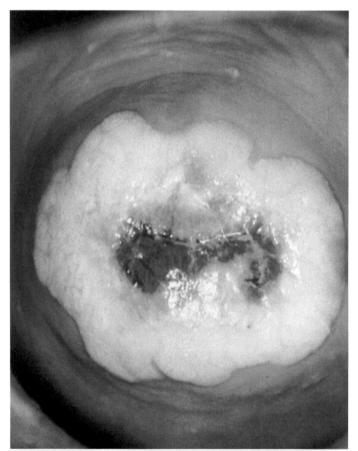

Fig. 6.91 Condyloma with marked keratinization. The keratin layer is so thick that a fissured surface is retained only focally, on the left side.

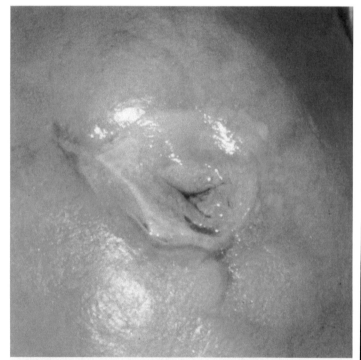

Fig. 6.92 Markedly keratinized flat condyloma surrounding the external os. Note the characteristic pearly, flat surface.

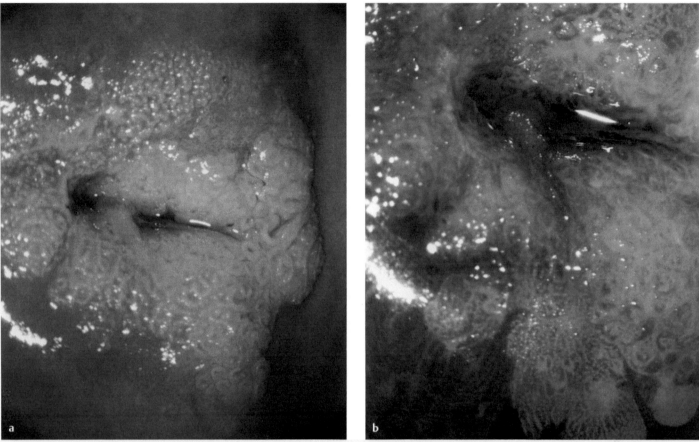

Fig. 6.93 **(a)** Flat to distinctly elevated condylomas around the external os and in the lower cervical canal. (Same patient as in Fig. 6.84, 6 months later.) **(b)** Iodine (Schiller's test) shows the typical patchy brown areas indicating glycogen storage in the condylomas. Histology showed LSIL (CIN 1) with koilocytosis.

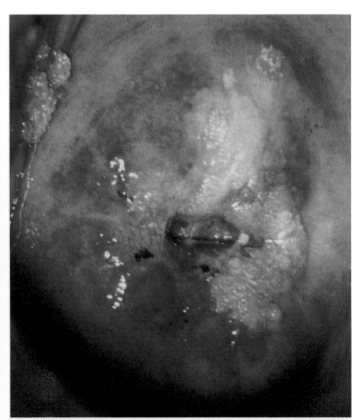

Fig. 6.94 Flat condylomas around the external os in an HIV-positive patient. Most of their surface is finely granular; some areas are smooth. Small condylomatous lesions dot the cervix and the vagina (HPV 16–positive).

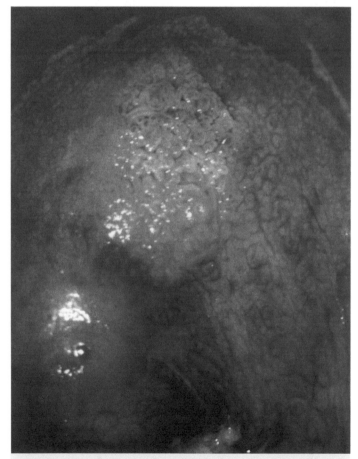

Fig. 6.95 Flat, fine papillary condylomatous excrescences within a mosaic. The mosaic is HPV 16–positive; histology showed LSIL (CIN 1).

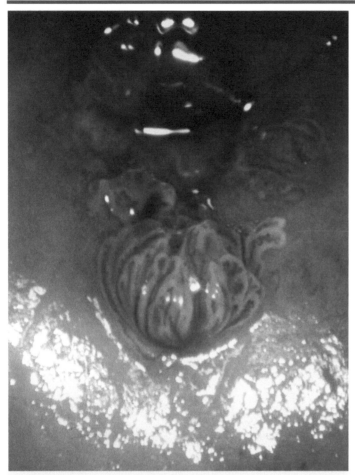

Fig. 6.96 Condyloma characterized by fingerlike processes with little keratinization.

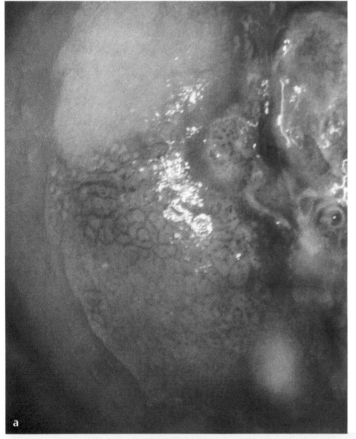

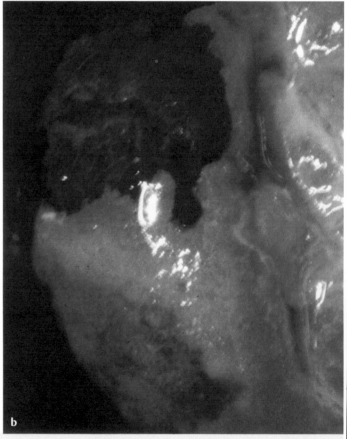

Fig. 6.97 (a) A shiny mother-of-pearl surface of a lesion also showing fine mosaic and punctation. Histologically, the white area corresponded to a flat condyloma, the mosaic showed LSIL (CIN 1). **(b)** After iodine (Schiller's test), the previously white lesion displays an iodine-positive mosaic. Histology showed flat condyloma. The mosaic and punctation, clearly visible before the Schiller's test, stain poorly. Less structured areas are light brown.

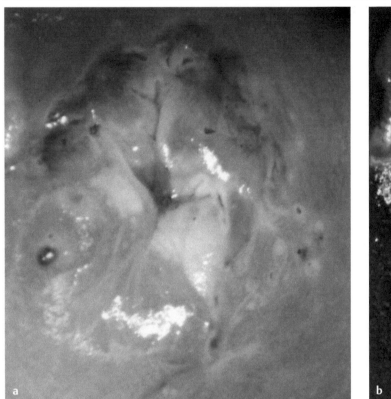
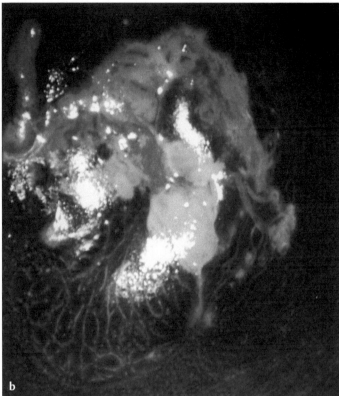

Fig. 6.98 (a) Shiny pearly lesion around the external os. The white epithelium was HSIL with koilocytosis. **(b)** The Schiller's test shows the other lesion and, beneath it, a fine iodine-positive mosaic.

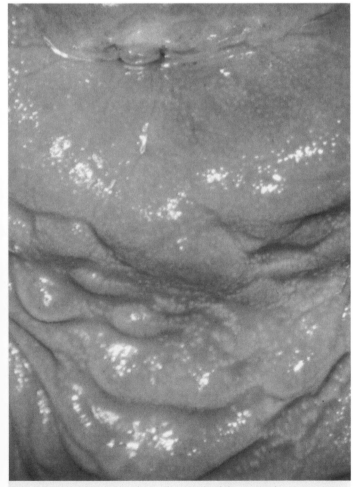

Fig. 6.99 Condylomatous colpitis. The cervix and the vagina show numerous white spots.

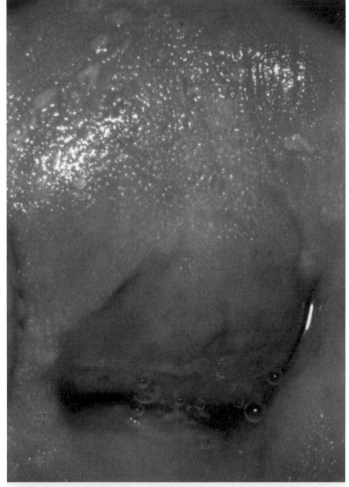

Fig. 6.100 Condylomatous vaginitis. There are circumscribed, slightly elevated condylomas within the granular area.

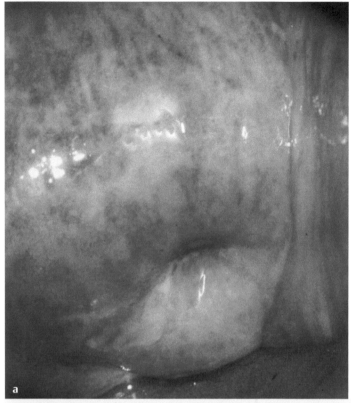

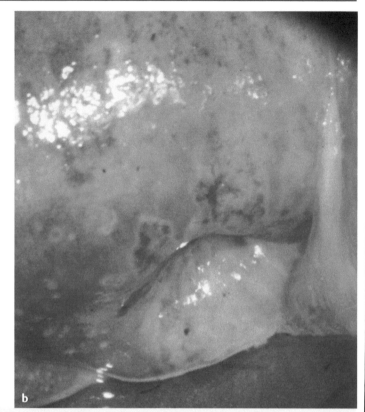

Fig. 6.101 (a) Irregular reddish stippling of the cervix from trichomonal infection. **(b)** The inflamed area becomes somewhat white to some extent after application of acetic acid; its margins are indistinct.

6.3.4 Inflammatory Changes

Diffuse inflammation of the vagina has a nonspecific colposcopic appearance. The appearance of focal lesions is of some significance because of their patchy inflammatory infiltration of the stroma accompanied by dilated capillaries. Diagnostic difficulties arise when such foci become bigger and indiscriminately arranged.

Trichomonal infection produces a typical frothy discharge. Removal of the secretions may reveal numerous red spots covering the cervix (Fig. 6.101a). The inflammatory foci vary in shape and in distribution. After application of acetic acid, the previously red areas turn whitish, the squamous epithelium being already loosened by the inflammation (Fig. 6.101b). The damaged epithelium can release its glycogen, with consequent failure to stain with iodine. Iodine typically imparts a leopard-skin appearance to inflammatory lesions (Fig. 6.102) and confirms the poor circumscription of larger lesions that might otherwise be mistaken for more serious abnormalities.

Colpitis macularis (strawberry cervix) has a unique colposcopic appearance, characterized by uniformly arranged red spots a few millimeters in size. It is usually due to *Trichomonas vaginalis* (Fig. 6.103a). The inflamed area is always iodine-negative, and its margin is indistinct (Fig. 6.103b). In severe cases, the vagina is also involved.

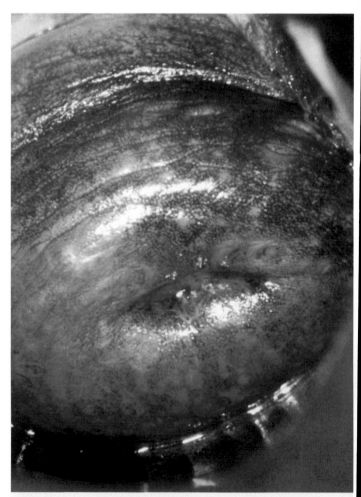

Fig. 6.102 The vague margins of the inflamed areas are well seen after application of iodine (Schiller's test).

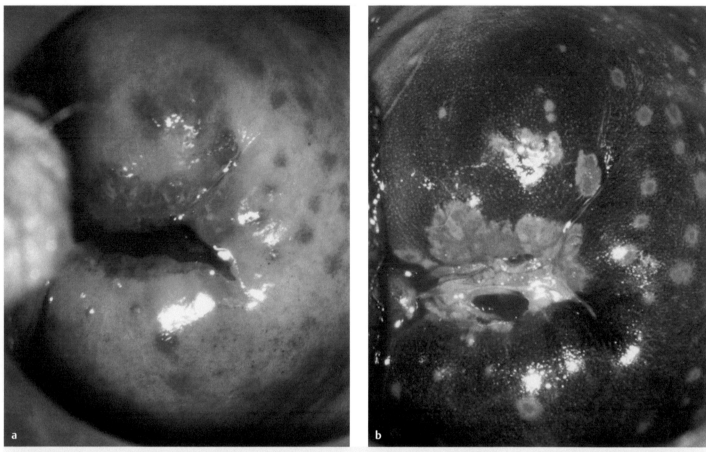

Fig. 6.103 (a) Colpitis macularis (strawberry cervix). Numerous round spots on the cervix and vagina are due to focal round cell infiltration. **(b)** After the Schiller's test, the inflamed areas are poorly demarcated and are separated by fields showing so-called condylomatous colpitis.

6.3.5 Polyps

Polyps are easily seen colposcopically, even if they are situated farther up in the endocervical canal. The aim of colposcopy is to detect them and evaluate their surface for signs of atypia. High polyps can be composed of columnar epithelium only, in which case the typical grapelike appearance will be seen. More often, the polyp is covered by smooth squamous epithelium (Figs. 6.104–6.109a, b). If the maturation of such histogenetically metaplastic squamous epithelium is irregular, then the various fields are clearly demarcated from each other (Figs. 6.105 and 6.106a, b). Rarely, the squamous epithelium is atypical; in such cases, the colposcopic changes conform to those that occur elsewhere on the cervix. Polyps can be single or multiple and can arise from ectopies, from TZs (Figs. 6.104, 6.106a, b, and 6.107), or from otherwise unremarkable cervices (Figs. 6.108 and 6.109a, b). On occasion, endometrial cancer can present as a bleeding polypoid mass protruding from the cervix (Fig. 6.110). A myoma in the statu nascendi is shown in Fig. 6.111.

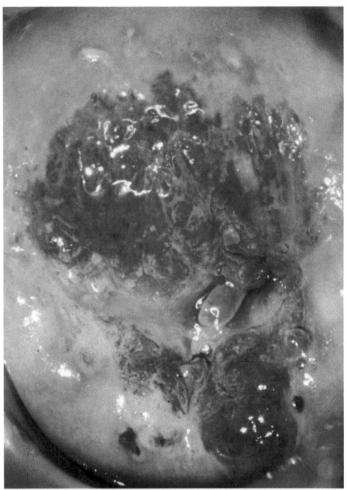

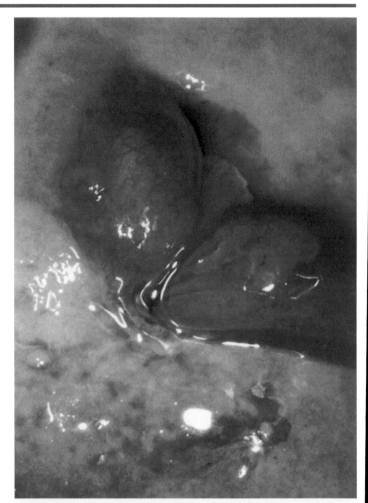

Fig. 6.104 Cervical polyp in the transformation zone. The polyp is covered by metaplastic squamous epithelium.

Fig. 6.105 Endocervical polyps that have undergone metaplasia. A nabothian follicle has developed within one of the polyps. The lowermost polyp shows that the metaplastic process developed in separate, well-defined fields.

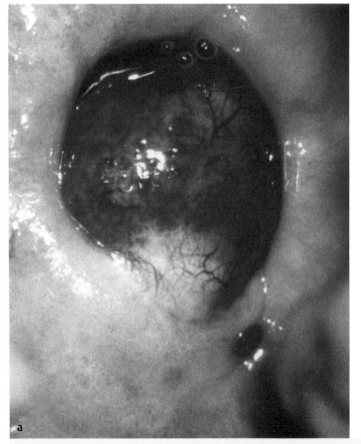

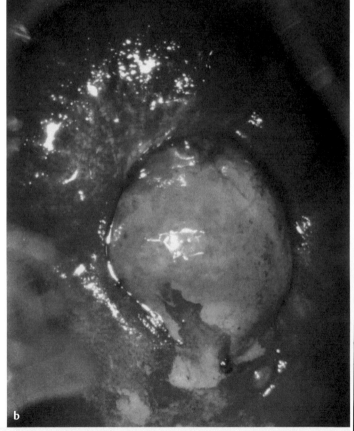

Fig. 6.106 (a) Broad-based polypoid structure corresponding to a nabothian follicle. **(b)** After application of iodine, the cervix stains brown and the nabothian follicle stains yellow.

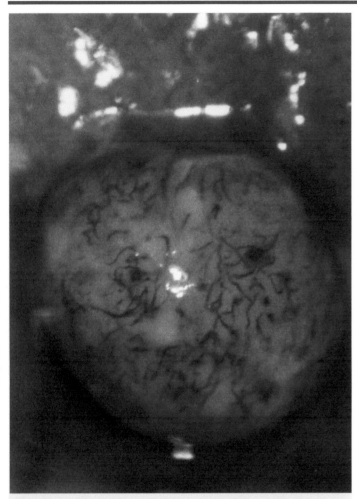

Fig. 6.107 Nabothian follicle with delicate nonsuspicious vessels on its surface.

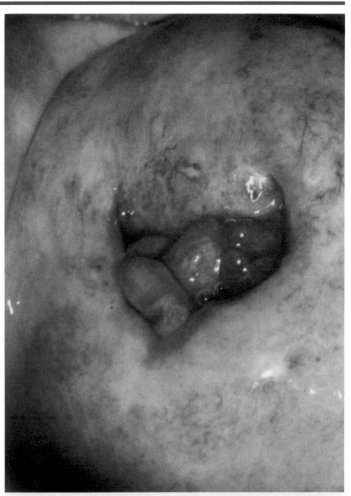

Fig. 6.108 Multiple polyps arising from an atrophic cervix. The metaplastic epithelium covering the polyps also arose in separate fields.

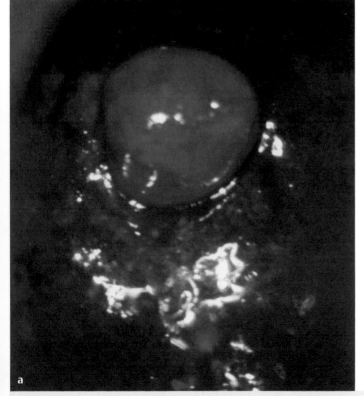

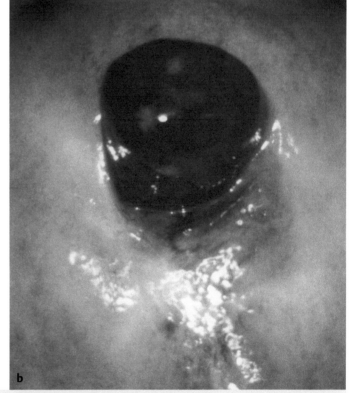

Fig. 6.109 (a) Polyp protruding from the external os. The surface is smooth and the origin unclear. (b) After application of iodine (Schiller's test), the cervix stains brown and the polyp stains yellow. Histology showed a cervical mucosal polyp with metaplastic epithelium.

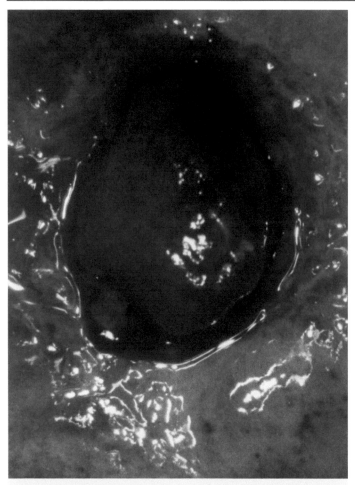

Fig. 6.110 Bleeding polyp protruding out of the cervical canal. The surface of the cervix shows signs of atrophy. Histology showed G1 endometrial carcinoma.

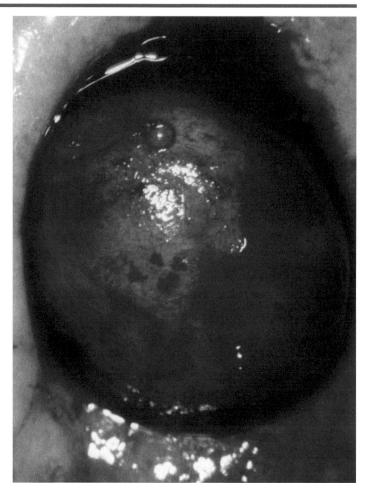

Fig. 6.111 Myoma in statu nascendi.

6.3.6 Postconization Changes

After conization, the cervix is usually smooth and covered by normal squamous epithelium. The SCJ is again situated at the external os. Occasionally, the scar after conization clearly stands out from the residual cervix (Fig. 6.112a) and can be mistaken for some other abnormality. However, with iodine (Schiller's test), the area in question stains brown like the rest of the cervix (Fig. 6.112b), and any nuance in color is due to scar tissue under the epithelium. This is a good example of how the stroma can influence the colposcopic appearance. Six weeks after conization, scarring can be extensive (Fig. 6.113).

The changes after loop conization are the same after cold-knife procedures. With correct technique, the entire SCJ is usually visible, which is helpful for follow-up colposcopy (Figs. 6.114 and 6.115). Laser vaporization techniques give excellent cosmetic results.

Residual lesions from incomplete excision by conization can be detected at follow-up colposcopy in the region of the reconstituted external os (Fig. 6.116). Sturmdorf's sutures for hemostasis after conization are obsolete, not only because they produce a poor cosmetic result.

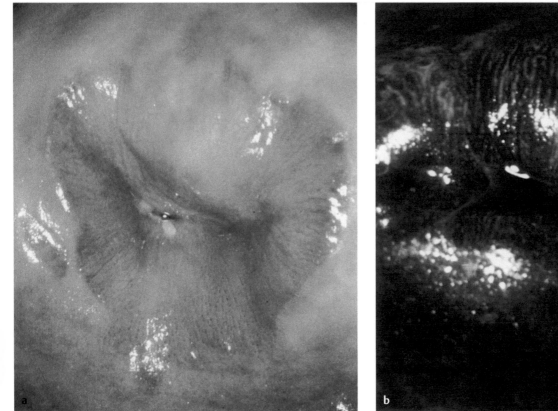
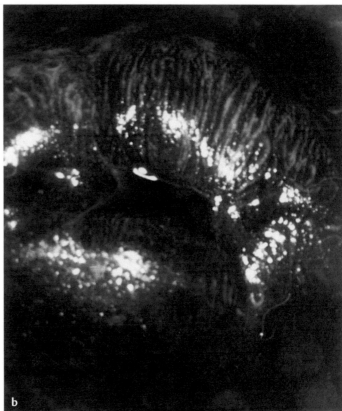

Fig. 6.112 **(a)** Cervix 1 year after conization. The excision site shows scarring and fine vasculature. **(b)** Iodine staining shows the uniform nature of the epithelium. The light yellow streaks correspond to scars.

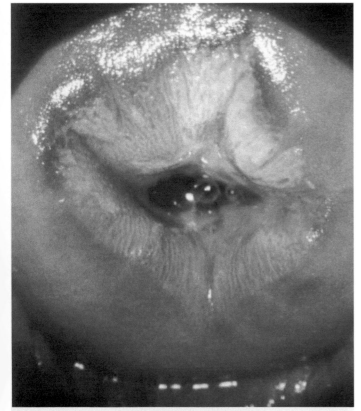

Fig. 6.113 Cervix 6 weeks after cold-knife conization. Scarring is clearly apparent. There is a small polyp in the cervical canal, and the squamocolumnar junction is visible in its entirety.

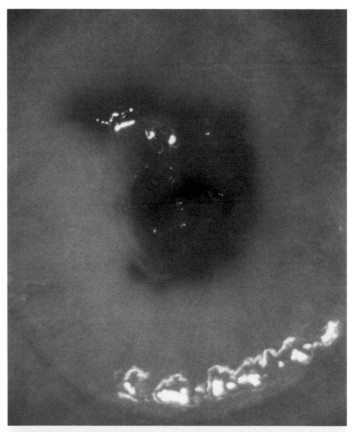

Fig. 6.114 Cervix 6 weeks after loop excision. A small scar can be seen. The squamocolumnar junction is visible in its entirety.

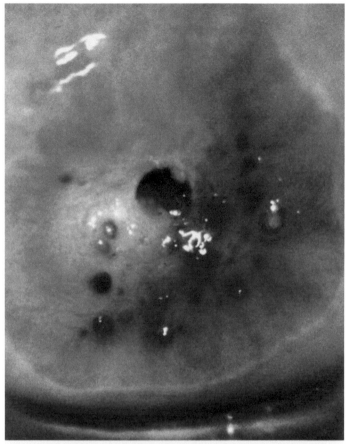

Fig. 6.115 Cervix 6 weeks after loop excision. There is slight scarring on the external os with somewhat increased scarring between 3 o'clock and 7 o'clock positions. Cervical glands with nonsuspicious vessels.

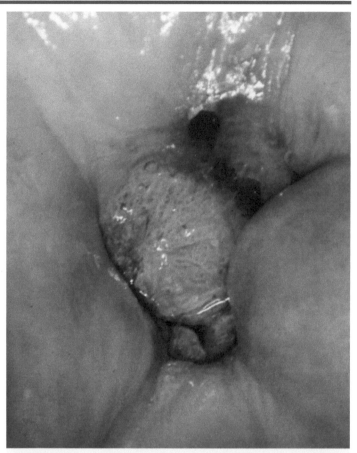

Fig. 6.116 The cervix after incomplete excision of HSIL (CIN 3) by conization. Note in the scar tissue an area of coarse punctation from residual dysplastic epithelium.

6.3.7 Changes Resulting from Prolapse

Prolapse results in exteriorization of the squamous epithelium of the cervix and portions of the vagina. The glycogen-containing squamous epithelium changes and becomes skin-like. Histology shows acanthosis and hyperkeratosis. This process proves that, according to demand, the nonkeratinized glycogen-containing epithelium can become like the epidermis, so-called *epidermization*. Colposcopically, we encounter far more often the *regenerative form* of metaplastic epithelium that arises from metaplasia in clearly defined fields and is of great colposcopic significance. The important difference between the reactive and regenerative types is the reversible nature of the former: after the stimulus ceases (i.e., after reduction of the prolapse), the epithelium resumes its original form. In contrast, the well-circumscribed regenerative type of metaplastic epithelium retains its position and contour. The regenerative type of metaplastic epithelium therefore is abnormal and in this respect resembles chronic dermatoses.

The colposcopic appearance of the epidermized cervix is reminiscent of skin both in color and in its wrinkled surface contour (Fig. 6.117). It is obvious even with the naked eye that this type of epithelium is tougher. A well-recognized complication of prolapse is ulceration of the extruded portion of the cervix or vagina. These ulcers are punched out, their floor is flat and usually very red (Fig. 6.118), but it can be dirty gray if superinfected. Ulcers caused by prolapse are not to be confused with cervical cancer coexisting with uterovaginal procidentia (Fig. 6.119).

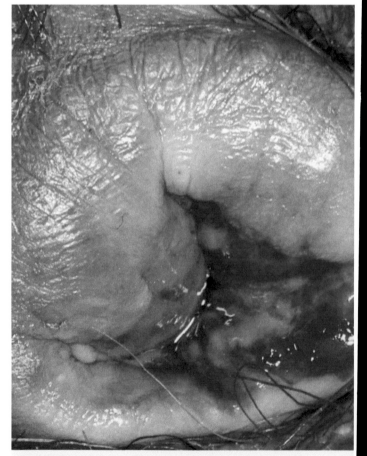

Fig. 6.117 Keratinization of uterovaginal prolapse. The ectocervical epithelium assumes the character of wrinkled skin.

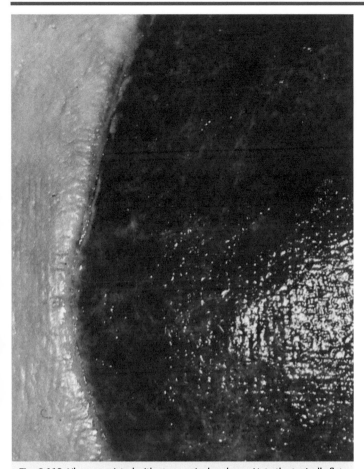

Fig. 6.118 Ulcer associated with uterovaginal prolapse. Note the typically flat floor and punched-out margin.

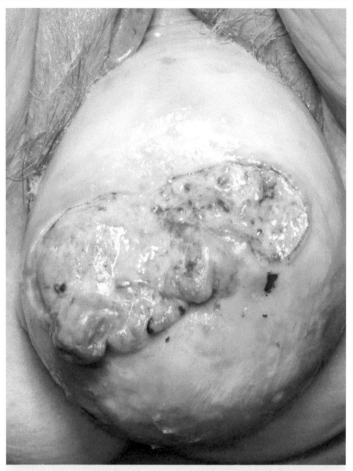

Fig. 6.119 Large cervical cancer in a patient with uterovaginal procidentia.

6.3.8 Endometriosis, Fistulas, Anatomic Anomalies

Endometriosis of the cervix is uncommon (Fig. 6.120). The posterior vaginal fornix is involved most frequently (Fig. 6.121). Endometriotic foci appear as bluish spots shimmering through the epithelium and are best seen before menstruation; they can disappear altogether during the proliferative phase of the cycle. Fistulas can occasionally develop in patients after surgery or radiation therapy of the lower genital tract.

Fistulas (Fig. 6.122) and anatomic anomalies such as septae (Fig. 6.123) can on occasion be documented at colposcopy.

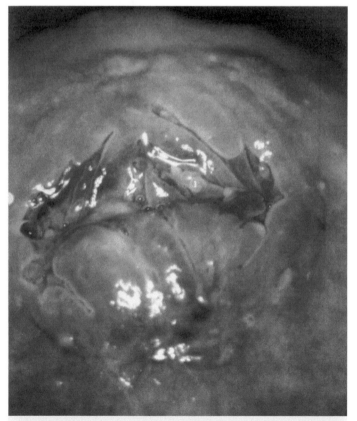

Fig. 6.120 Small bluish focus of endometriosis on the anterior lip at 2 o'clock position of a transformation zone with still recognizable rugae of the ectropion.

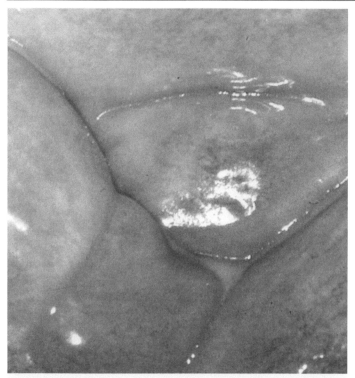

Fig. 6.121 Bluish endometriotic deposit in the posterior fornix of a 38-year-old woman on day 24 of the menstrual cycle.

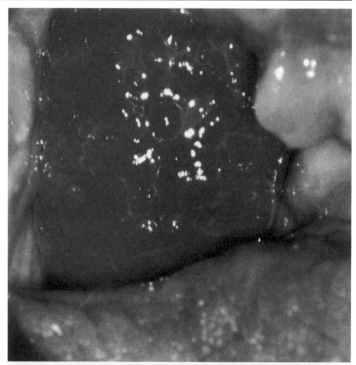

Fig. 6.122 Vesicovaginal fistula after primary radiation treatment for carcinoma of the cervix. The bladder mucosa is red and grapelike without the application of acetic acid.

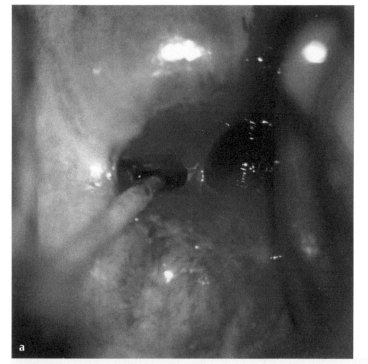

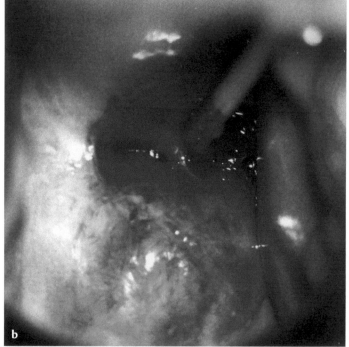

Fig. 6.123 Transformation zone in a cervix divided by a septum. The probe is in the left **(a)** and right **(b)** part of the cervical canal.

6.4 Assessment of Colposcopic Findings

Colposcopists want to predict the histology underlying colposcopic findings. This is straightforward as far as original squamous epithelium, ectopy, or normal TZ are concerned. The task becomes more difficult when colposcopic findings are abnormal and the question arises whether they are benign or neoplastic. It is challenging when normal and abnormal colposcopic findings differ only in subtle features.

It is important to appreciate that no colposcopic findings are pathognomonic of malignancy. In practice, the colposcopist must distinguish between two patterns: *nonsuspicious findings* and *suspicious findings*. With experience, the colposcopist will succeed increasingly in distinguishing between the two, thereby reducing the number of biopsies. *Suspicious findings* are not synonymous with *abnormal findings* because the latter are not always due to premalignant lesions.

6.4.1 Benign Metaplastic Epithelium and Squamous Intraepithelial Neoplasia

Variations in the interpretation of colposcopic findings are due to the fact that colposcopy is often carried out only to evaluate patients with abnormal smears. Patient selection thus ensures that in most cases abnormal colposcopic findings correspond to histologically atypical epithelia. Those who use colposcopy routinely take a different view. They appreciate that the histologic counterparts of leukoplakia, punctation, mosaic, or acetowhite epithelium are more often due to metaplastic than to dysplastic epithelia.

Metaplastic epithelium is a great imitator. It arises in the TZ. The metaplastic process can result in normal, mature squamous epithelium; immature, metaplastic epithelium; or SIL. Like the epidermis, metaplastic epithelium is composed mostly of prickle cells and shows at least parakeratosis. It is important for colposcopic diagnosis because metaplastic epithelium can develop in clearly demarcated fields. Normal glycogen-containing epithelium can also change to diffusely keratinizing metaplastic epithelium, as in prolapse.

If the metaplastic epithelium is focal, the individual fields have sharp borders. The surface usually shows parakeratosis or hyperkeratosis. Also, metaplastic epithelium is often peg-forming, being subdivided by tall stromal papillae. The pegs can appear as isolated columns or be arranged in interlacing netlike ridges.

Metaplastic epithelium can therefore appear in the TZ as leukoplakia, punctation, mosaic, or even acetowhite epithelium.

6.5 Criteria for Differential Diagnosis

The differential diagnosis of colposcopic findings is based on a number of features:
- Sharp borders.
- Response to acetic acid (white epithelium).
- Surface contour.
- Appearance of gland openings.
- Appearance of blood vessels.
- Surface area (size).
- Combinations of abnormalities.
- Iodine uptake.
- Keratinization.

6.5.1 Sharp Borders

Sharp borders are among the most important colposcopic findings but often underappreciated in the colposcopic and pathology-literature. Almost all colposcopically significant lesions have sharp borders. Such borders are also found within large lesions, especially after the application of iodine (Schiller's test).

Any sharply circumscribed epithelium has developed via transformation. Reactive changes, such as those induced by inflammation, are usually diffuse. Sharp borders are often recognizable by native colposcopy. In any case, they become distinct after application of acetic acid iodine (Fig. 6.124). In contrast to punctation and mosaic, which are always sharply circumscribed, punctation from inflammation and mosaic simulated by chance arrangement of blood vessels have indistinct margins. In most cases, the criterion of sharp borders alone enables one to distinguish between significant and nonspecific colposcopic lesions. This feature, however, cannot be used to differentiate between metaplastic epithelia and SIL because both have sharp borders.

6.5.2 Response to Acetic Acid (White Epithelium)

Application of acetic acid clarifies the colposcopic appearance by removing mucus. Acetic acid also induces swelling of SIL because of its poor intercellular cohesiveness. At the same time, the color of the epithelium changes from red to white. If, in addition, the lesion shows punctation or mosaic, the white epithelial fields project above the surface. Vascular structures remain red and consequently become better contrasted. The atypical TZ remains unstructured except for the gland openings and thus displays a white surface (Fig. 6.33). This feature is called "white epithelium" if neither mosaic nor punctation is present. The cohesiveness of the epithelium is directly proportional to its differentiation, the effect of acetic acid being maximal on undifferentiated epithelium. Thus, its effect on mildly dysplastic epithelium is considerably less than on HSIL (Figs. 6.125 and 6.126). Condylomata, especially flat ones, show a characteristic shiny white mother-of-pearl hue (Figs. 6.91 and 6.93a).

6.5.3 Surface Contour

Punctation and mosaic produced by metaplastic epithelium resemble a delicate sketch, the dots being small and the lines fine. The distance between the spots is not excessive, and the epithelial fields between the lines are small and regular. These features become more distinct after application of acetic acid (Fig. 6.127) but do not project from the surface. Punctation produced by SIL can appear in marked cases (HSIL) as *elevated papillae* (Fig. 6.128) and the lines of mosaic as *coarse ridges* (Fig. 6.126). In contrast to metaplastic epithelium, the dots (or papillae) of SIL are more widely separated; similarly, the epithelial cobbles of a mosaic are larger. After application of acetic acid, these structures become more prominent and raised above the surface. In clear-cut cases, it is easy to differentiate between fine and coarse mosaics and punctations. There is a spectrum of appearances between the two extremes, the proper categorization of which depends on the evaluation of the remaining criteria.

Flat condylomas, which are essentially benign, can show coarse patterns of punctation and mosaic with an irregular surface

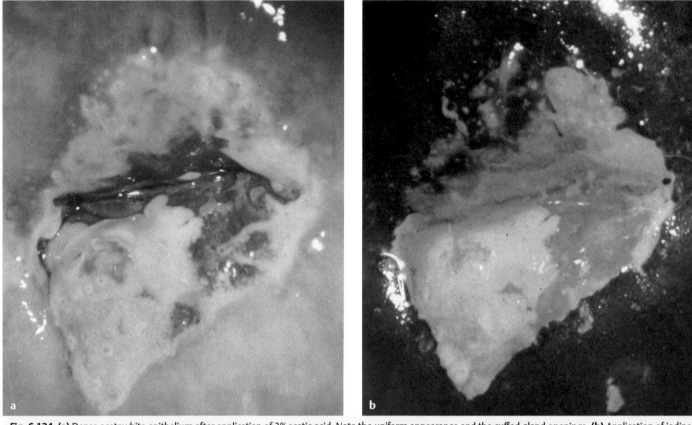

Fig. 6.124 **(a)** Dense acetowhite epithelium after application of 3% acetic acid. Note the uniform appearance and the cuffed gland openings. **(b)** Application of iodine reveals that the typically yellowish discoloration is focal and the sharp border segmental. Between the 9 o'clock and 12 o'clock positions, the margin is quite indistinct. Histology of the iodine-yellow area returned HSIL (CIN 3).

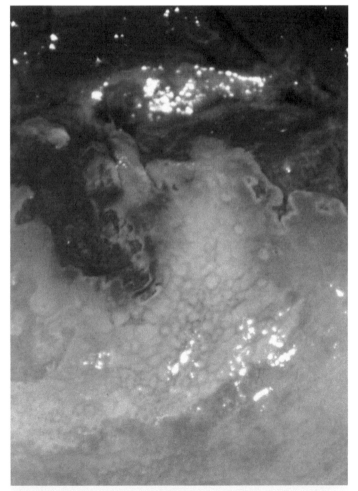

Fig. 6.125 Moderately coarse mosaic with mild accentuation of the surface contour following application of acetic acid. Histology showed HSIL (CIN 2).

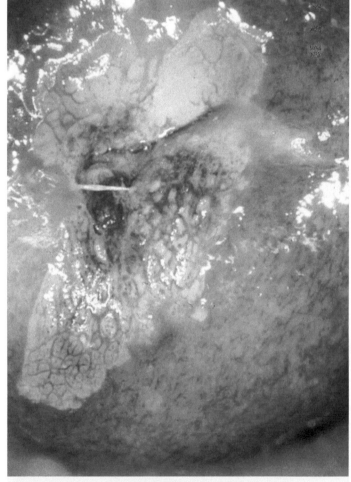

Fig. 6.126 Coarse mosaic with marked swelling and elevation of the epithelium after application of acetic acid. Histology showed HSIL (CIN 3).

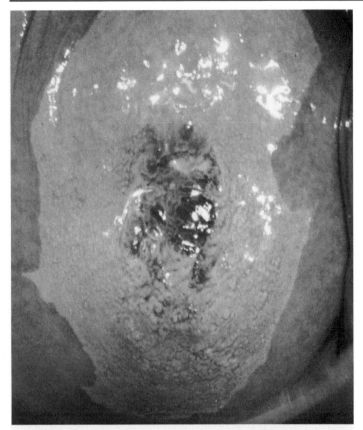

Fig. 6.127 Fairly fine mosaic. The sharply circumscribed acetowhite epithelium remains in the same plane as its surroundings. Histology showed metaplastic epithelium.

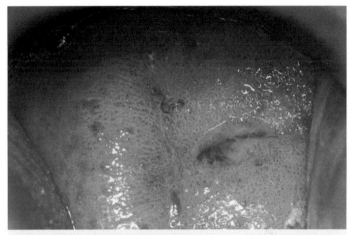

Fig. 6.128 Pronounced papillary punctation. Histology showed HSIL (CIN 3) with early stromal invasion (FIGO stage IA1).

configuration (Fig. 6.129). Their pearly surface can distinguish them from HSIL, the surfaces of which are characteristically opaque. Because flat condylomas frequently coexist with papillary or spiked condylomas, the presence of one or more spikes on or near the lesion is a useful diagnostic feature.

6.5.4 Cuffed Gland Openings

The presence of gland openings is a characteristic feature of the TZ. They are visible proof that columnar epithelium has been replaced by squamous epithelium. The metaplasia is often restricted to the rims of the gland outlets, leaving the mouths open. The metaplasia can also involve the glandular crypts, so that the gland openings will be completely lined by squamous epithelium. Colposcopically, such events are evidenced by the development of white cuffs after application of acetic acid (Fig. 6.19). The cuff will be wider and more pronounced after acetic acid (Fig. 6.33) in HSIL compared with normal or metaplastic epithelium (Figs. 6.19 and 6.23). Such an appearance is referred to as a "cuffed gland opening."

6.5.5 Blood Vessels

Over the years, a great deal of importance has been attached to the vascular pattern. The nature of the blood vessels is an important diagnostic feature. During the reproductive years, the vasculature is not always visible under the well-developed squamous epithelium. The vascular pattern is enhanced by inflammation and by the attenuation of the covering epithelium and is a prominent feature of well-circumscribed epithelial lesions.

The blood vessels are best inspected at the beginning of the colposcopic examination. Acetic acid can suppress the vasculature

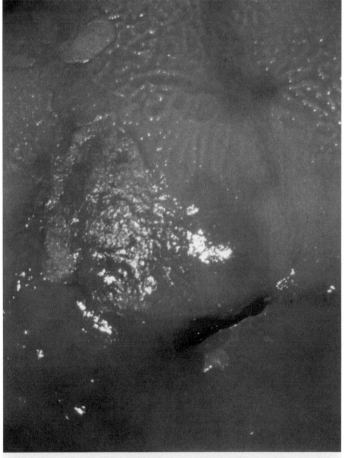

Fig. 6.129 Numerous flat condylomas with gyrated surfaces. In between, there are small, markedly cornified areas.

to the point that it almost disappears (Fig. 6.27). A green filter, which screens out red and makes the vessels appear dark, can enhance the vascular appearance. Like others, we distinguish between various vascular patterns.

6.5.6 Nonsuspicious Vascular Pattern

The course and branching of the vessels are regular, with gradual reduction in caliber. The distance between the regular terminal capillary loops, the so-called *intercapillary distance*, is normal (Fig. 6.130a–f). The distribution of these vessels is usually diffuse, and they do not appear in lesions that are clearly circumscribed. Nonsuspicious vessels are characteristic of diffuse inflammation, when the cervix assumes a stippled appearance. On higher magnification, the capillary loops are hairpin or, when not seen in their entirety, comma-shaped.

Diagnostic difficulties can arise if the inflammatory foci are not regularly dispersed, as in colpitis macularis, but vary in size and distribution (Fig. 6.101). The blood vessels in such lesions can be particularly clearly etched out and can be fork-shaped or antler-shaped; the intercapillary distance, however, remains normal. The appearances can mimic punctation. These lesions are always poorly circumscribed, a feature seen especially well after application of iodine.

The neat, finely knit meshwork of blood vessels of atrophic, postmenopausal squamous epithelium can be distinctive (Fig. 6.131).

The individual vessels of the vascular network of the normal TZ tend to be long and regularly arborizing, with no abrupt change in direction or in caliber. The vessels decrease in caliber as they branch out. Nabothian follicles show normal vascular patterns. The long blood vessels that traverse these yellowish structures are relatively large and show regular branching and gradual loss of caliber (Fig. 6.132). They are so characteristic that the presence of deep-seated and otherwise invisible nabothian follicles can be inferred (Fig. 6.133).

6.5.7 Suspicious Vascular Pattern

The first hint of atypia is the presence of blood vessels in sharply circumscribed areas (especially with iodine) (Fig. 6.130g, h). The blood vessels in punctation are fine to coarse and hairpin, comma, or tortuous (corkscrew) in shape, but still regularly arranged. Within this pattern, the appearances show wide variation. The capillary loops in punctation resulting from metaplastic epithelium are delicate and regular, with no increase in the intercapillary distance (Fig. 6.133). The tortuous corkscrew and comma-shaped vessels associated with SIL are coarser, show haphazard branching, and vary in caliber; the intercapillary distance is increased (Figs. 6.134–6.136).

A similar range of appearances is seen in the various expressions of mosaic. The delicate mosaic pattern associated with metaplastic epithelium is produced by small, evenly distributed epithelial fields subdivided by thin red ridges (Fig. 6.127). In coarse mosaic, the dividing lines are more definite, the resulting fields larger and more irregular (Fig. 6.126).

Even relatively regular and more or less parallel vessels can appear suspicious when they are wider (compare Figs. 6.131 and 6.137) and show an abrupt change in caliber (Fig. 6.134). The vascular pattern can on occasion mimic a mosaic. Closer inspection, however, shows that the vessels in these circumstances display treelike branching and uniform reduction in caliber and appear in poorly circumscribed areas (Fig. 6.130f).

Atypical Vessels

The 2011 colposcopic terminology includes atypical vessels as a separate diagnostic entity. Atypical vessels show a completely irregular and haphazard disposition, great variation in caliber, and abrupt changes in direction, often forming acute angles (Fig. 6.130i–k). The intercapillary distance is increased and tends to be variable (Fig. 6.138). Highly atypical vessels are characteristic of invasive carcinomas (Figs. 6.69b, 6.139, and 6.140). When flattish lesions display focal collections of such vessels, microinvasion should be suspected (Fig. 6.141).

6.5.8 Surface Area (Size)

Morphometric studies of conization specimens have shown that the surface extent of SIL increases with the severity of the lesion. Thus, lesions caused by ESI are larger than those from HSIL, which in turn are larger than those from LSIL. This does not mean that fields of HSIL are larger than those of LSIL per se but that the former are more likely to be combined with the latter so that the total area is larger. The marked increase in the surface extent of early invasive lesions is also due to coalescence of fields of LSIL and HSIL. There is a direct relationship between size and likelihood of invasion.

The same conclusions apply to colposcopic lesions. Colposcopically suspicious but small lesions are frequently not of histologic significance, whereas colposcopically highly suspicious lesions are consistently extensive. Small lesions are more likely to be LSIL than HSIL or invasive carcinoma. This does not contradict the principles of evaluation of intraepithelial lesions as detailed in Chapter 1. On the contrary, the coexistence of different epithelia shows that invasive potential is acquired by their coalescence and not by progression of one type to another.

These statements do not apply to metaplastic epithelium, which can involve only small areas or cover the whole cervix and even parts of the vagina (congenital TZ). Consequently, size alone is not a diagnostic criterion; size should be considered only in concert with other criteria. If the latter point to atypia, large size should further raise the index of suspicion. This has been accounted for in the 2011 nomenclature (see Chapter 5) with the inclusion of the size of the lesion (expressed as the number of cervical quadrants or percentage of the cervix covered).

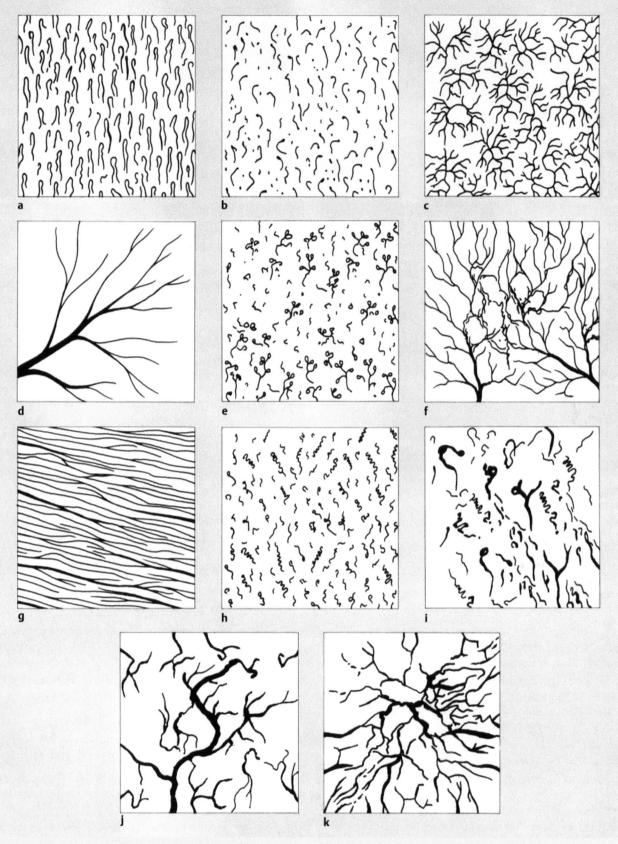

Fig. 6.130 Normal and atypical vascular patterns on the cervix. **(a)** Hairpin-shaped capillary loops. **(b)** Comma-shaped capillaries. **(c)** Blood vessels with regular branching. **(d)** Long, regularly branching vascular tree, with gradual decrease in caliber. **(e)** Staghorn-like vessels, seen especially in inflammation. **(f)** Regular vascular network, simulating mosaic. **(g)** Long parallel-coursing blood vessels, with some variation in caliber. **(h)** Irregular corkscrew vessels that vary only slightly in caliber. **(i)** Bizarre, tortuous, atypical vessels, with marked variation in caliber. **(j)** Atypical blood vessels with gross variation in caliber and arrangement and abrupt changes in direction. **(k)** Irregular vessels with great fluctuation in caliber.

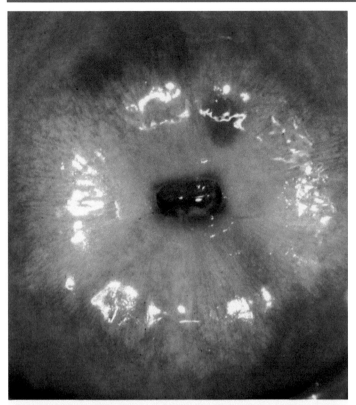

Fig. 6.131 Thin, atrophic squamous epithelium allows the fine radial network of blood vessels to shine through; the vascular pattern is not suspicious (compare with Fig. 6.12).

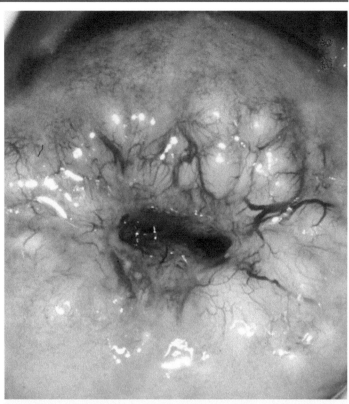

Fig. 6.132 Typical vascular tree over a nabothian follicle. Note the regular branching.

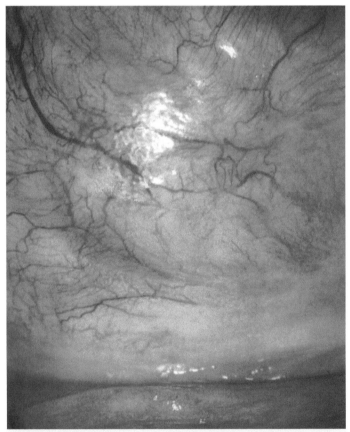

Fig. 6.133 Long, regularly branching blood vessels over the surface of a deep nabothian follicle. Note the gradual decrease in caliber.

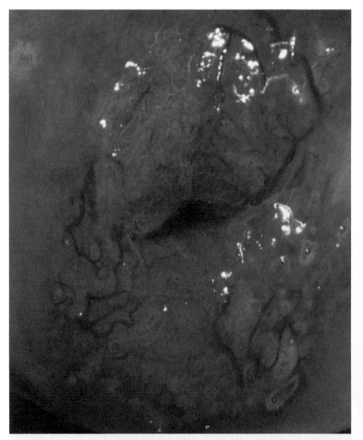

Fig. 6.134 Long, suspicious vessels in white epithelium. The caliber of the vessels varies slightly, and there are some abrupt changes in direction. Histology showed LSIL (CIN 1) with koilocytosis.

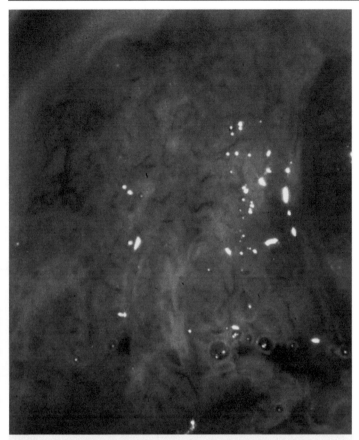

Fig. 6.135 Suspicious vessels in a white epithelium. Histology showed HSIL (CIN 3).

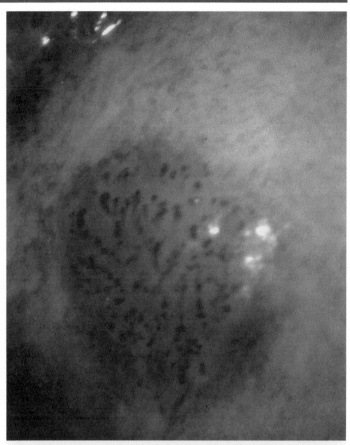

Fig. 6.136 Atypical vessels. The coarse, tortuous, comma-shaped, and corkscrew-shaped vessels vary distinctly in caliber. The intercapillary distance is markedly increased. Histology showed HSIL with early stromal invasion (FIGO stage IA1).

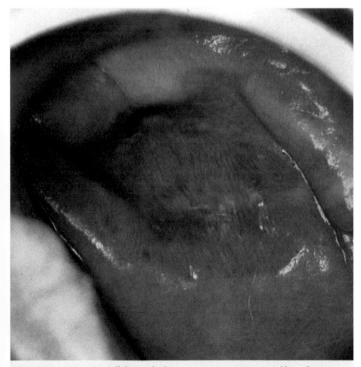

Fig. 6.137 Coarse parallel vessels showing great variation in caliber, skirting an invasive squamous cell carcinoma.

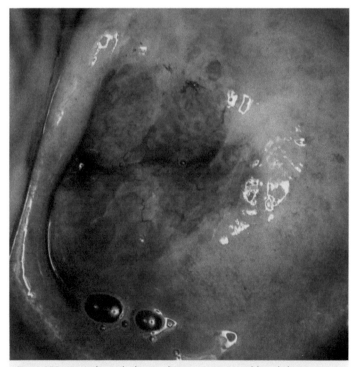

Fig. 6.138 Atypical vessels showing large variation in width and abrupt changes in direction at the margin of a squamous cell carcinoma in the canal.

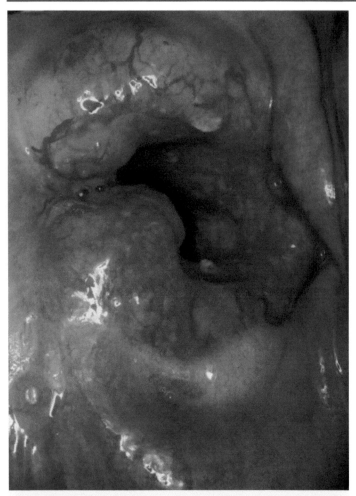

Fig. 6.139 Highly atypical vessels on the anterior lip in a partly exophytic and partly endophytic squamous cell carcinoma. Note the complete irregularity and large variations in width.

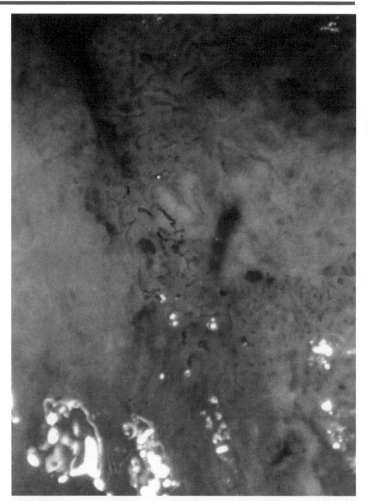

Fig. 6.140 A great variety of atypical vessels in an invasive squamous cell carcinoma.

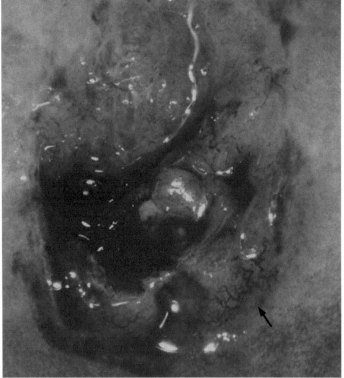

Fig. 6.141 Focal collection of atypical vessels over the surface of a microcarcinoma on the posterior lip (arrow).

6.6 Combinations of Abnormalities

Table 6.1 lists the rate of SIL or microinvasion in cone biopsies according to types of abnormal colposcopic findings. The rate of SIL or microinvasion is less than 50% for all types of individual findings; but if the patterns of leukoplakia, mosaic, and punctation are combined, the chance of finding SIL or microinvasion rises to 80%. These facts are entirely consistent with the observation that significant lesions are a patchwork of several epithelial types, including those showing various degrees of atypia.

6.6.1 Iodine Uptake

Colposcopic findings differ markedly in the intensity of staining with iodine (Lugol's solution; Schiller's test). Also, iodine staining enhances colposcopic borders. Brownish or brown staining from glycogen decreases the risk of SIL or invasive disease (Fig. 6.142a, b). An area that does not take up iodine at all can contain columnar epithelium or thin, regenerating, nonspecific epithelium. Well-developed metaplastic epithelium characteristically stains uniformly canary yellow and remains flat (Fig. 6.143). SIL also stains canary yellow, but it becomes mottled, and its surface is not so smooth. In cases of punctation and mosaic, the surface contour remains more clearly visible when the epithelium is dysplastic and not metaplastic, as the latter is essentially flat. The same applies when the Schiller's test is used.

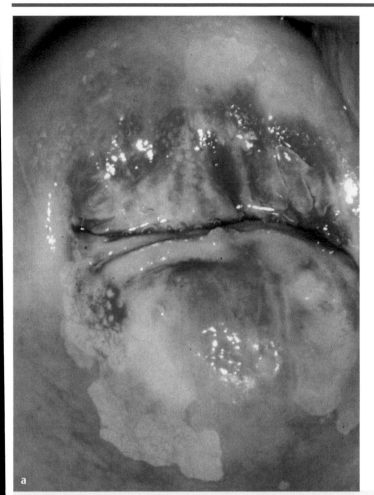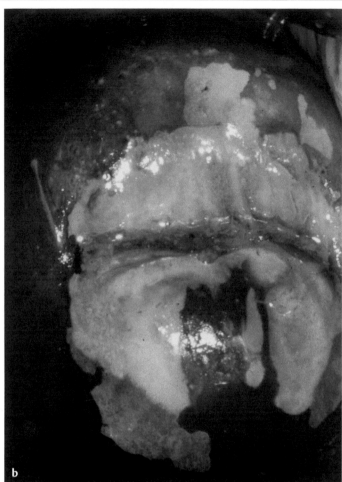

Fig. 6.142 **(a)** Acetic acid reveals a raised lesion with a variegated appearance between 6 o'clock and 8 o'clock (so-called ridge sign). Between 3 o'clock and 6 o'clock are two distinct fields of acetowhite epithelium (so-called inner border sign). Note the moderately coarse mosaic between 8 o'clock and 9 o'clock. **(b)** Iodine staining allows a more detailed analysis of an already complex colposcopic picture. The area seen in (a), now brownish, is probably a flat condyloma. The brown area on the posterior lip represents fully mature transformed squamous epithelium. The equally well-demarcated iodine-yellow area at 12 o'clock is due to metaplastic epithelium. The remaining yellow patches are HSIL (CIN 3).

Table 6.1 Colposcopic findings and corresponding histology in 118 patients with SIL (CIN) who underwent conization

Colposcopic findings	HSIL (CIN 2/3) or microinvasion	LSIL (CIN 1)
Nonsuspicious iodine-yellow area	0%	6%
Mosaic or punctation inside the TZ	76%	4%
Mosaic or punctation outside the TZ	20%	9%
Acetowhite epithelium	76%	4%
Leukoplakia	30%	8%

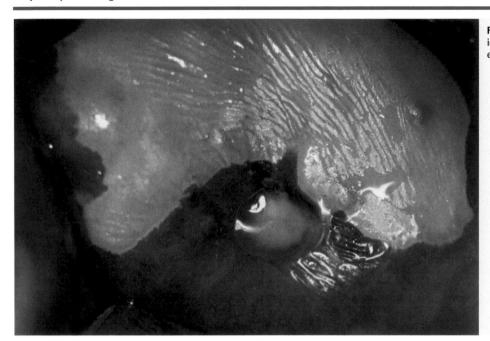

Fig. 6.143 Sharply circumscribed, smooth, iodine-yellow lesion from metaplastic squamous epithelium.

6.6.2 Keratinization

Keratinization is not a particularly useful diagnostic criterion. All grades of keratinization, from mild parakeratosis to pronounced hyperkeratosis, both of which appear colposcopically as leukoplakia, can be seen with both metaplastic epithelium and SIL. However, a mild degree of keratinization often corresponds to metaplastic epithelium, whereas flaky keratin suggests atypia.

The keratin layer obscures not only the surface contour but also the margins, and inhibits the effect of acetic acid. There is poor uptake of iodine resulting in a light yellow color. If the keratin layer can be peeled off, features of diagnostic importance may emerge. All cases of leukoplakia should be evaluated by biopsy.

6.6.3 Weighing Differential Diagnostic Criteria

The diagnostic features described in this chapter can be expressed to varying degrees and can be found singly or in combination. The more distinct a feature is and the greater the variety of features seen in combination, the higher the index of suspicion. Lesions should be viewed with a degree of suspicion by beginners, who should evaluate their findings by biopsy as part of the learning process. Quality can also be improved by repeating the smear if it was initially negative. With increasing practice, the colposcopist will be able to distinguish between benign and suspicious findings with some confidence. However, colposcopy cannot reliably distinguish between various forms of intraepithelial neoplasia.

Further Reading

Bornstein J, Bentley J, Bösze P, et al. 2011 colposcopic terminology of the International Federation for Cervical Pathology and Colposcopy. Obstet Gynecol 2012;120(1):166–172

Fritsch H, Hoermann R, Bitsche M, Pechriggl E, Reich O. Development of epithelial and mesenchymal regionalization of the human fetal utero-vaginal anlagen. J Anat 2013;222(4):462–472

Girardi F. The topography of abnormal colposcopy findings. Cervix 1993;11:45–52

Meisels A, Fortin R, Roy M. Condylomatous lesions of the cervix. II. Cytologic, coplposcopic and histopathologic study. Acta Cytol 1977;21:379-390

Wright VC. Colposcopy of adenocarcinoma in situ and adenocarcinoma of the uterine cervix: differentiation from other cervical lesions. J Low Genit Tract Dis 1999;3(2):83–97

Chapter 7

Colposcopy in Pregnancy

7

7 Colposcopy in Pregnancy

A gynecologic examination is indicated in early pregnancy if the patient has not recently had one. This should include a Pap smear and, we believe, colposcopy. The scenario of cervical cancers diagnosed in pregnancy (usually in women without standard gynecologic care) has become uncommon.

The most prominent colposcopic finding seen in pregnancy is the increase in size and number of the blood vessels, leading to hyperemia of the cervix. The stroma is softened and edematous, and the cervix becomes enlarged. The endocervical mucosa is hyperplastic. Proliferation of the columnar cells leads to enlargement and ramification of the glandular crypts, with formation of numerous secondary clefts and tunnels. The endocervical mucosa becomes velvety as a result of deeper extension into the stroma. The end result is a honeycomb appearance of the gland field.

Another characteristic change in pregnancy is a decidual reaction of the stroma. This can be limited and focal or quite extensive and can on occasion produce polypoid lesions referred to as *decidual polyps* (Figs. 7.1–7.3).

An ectocervix completely covered by squamous epithelium will not change much during the course of the pregnancy. However, occasionally, a pregnant woman can develop ectopy, or a preexisting ectopy can increase in size as a result of the increased volume of the cervix. (Outside pregnancy ectopy does not develop de novo.) It is also possible to produce pseudoectopy during the later stages of pregnancy by everting the cervical lips during speculum examination.

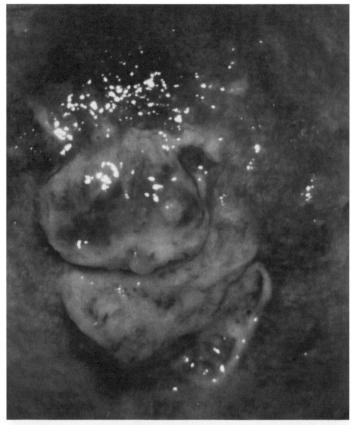

Fig. 7.1 Gravida 3, 20 weeks' gestation. Deciduosis. Grayish, solid formation at the external os. The formation is covered by fibrin, not epithelium. Histology showed a decidual reaction of the stroma.

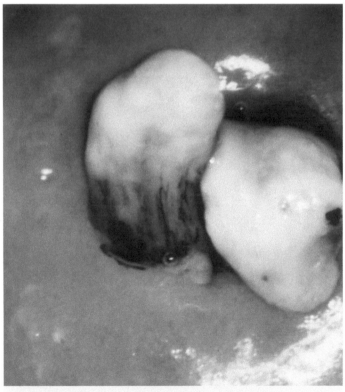

Fig. 7.2 Gravida 2, 8 weeks' gestation. Two decidual polyps in the cervical canal. Their surface is covered with fibrin, which obscures the epithelium. Note the vascular pattern, which is typical for decidual polyps.

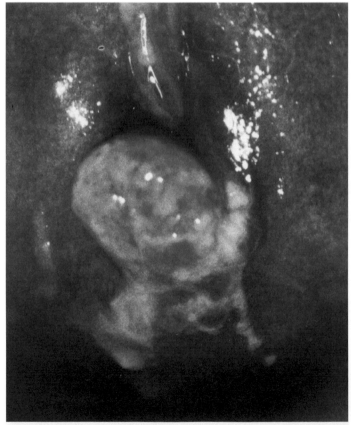

Fig. 7.3 Gravida 2, 16 weeks' gestation, decidual polyp in the cervical canal. The cervix is livid.

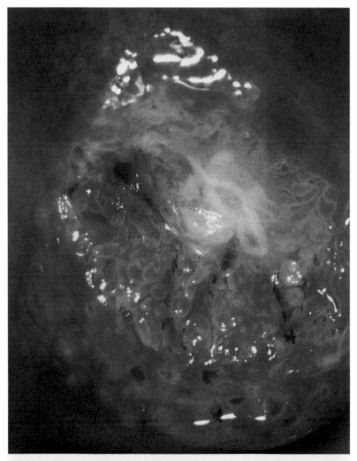

Fig. 7.4 Gravida 3, 17 weeks' gestation. Ectopy with a coarsened texture and deep longitudinal folds. On the posterior lip, transformation is complete, with gland openings and small nabothian cysts shining through. Livid coloration of the entire cervical mucosa. In the os, there is viscous mucus with whitish threads and granules typical of pregnancy.

The cervical mucus undergoes characteristic changes during pregnancy, becoming viscous and cloudy, whitish or yellowish, and containing threads or particles (Figs. 7.4 and 7.5). The mucus can be more difficult to remove with acetic acid than in the nonpregnant patient.

Apart from lesions such as decidual polyps (Fig. 7.1), there are no colposcopic findings specific for pregnancy. The changes occurring during pregnancy are the same as those described in Chapter 6. The same applies to reactive changes, inflammation, and infections.

In the past, there has been lively debate as to whether squamous intraepithelial lesion (SIL; also known as cervical intraepithelial neoplasia [CIN]) can develop during pregnancy and regress after the puerperium. Of course, low-grade squamous intraepithelial lesion (LSIL) can regress independently of pregnancy. In contrast, a number of studies have shown that high-grade squamous intraepithelial lesion (HSIL; CIN 3) detected during pregnancy does not regress postpartum. Systematic examination of the cervices of women in early pregnancy has even shown a surprisingly high incidence of persisting HSIL (CIN 3). These results are of interest from the epidemiologic point of view and underline the importance of standard gynecologic care during pregnancy.

7.1 Effects of Pregnancy on Colposcopic Findings

Lividity of the cervicovaginal mucosa was a clinical sign of pregnancy long before ultrasound and immunologic tests were developed. Lividity is due to the increased vascularity of the pelvic organs, especially the venous plexuses. Marked fluid retention gives the cervix a soft consistency, and it becomes softer as the pregnancy advances. Increased fragility and a tendency

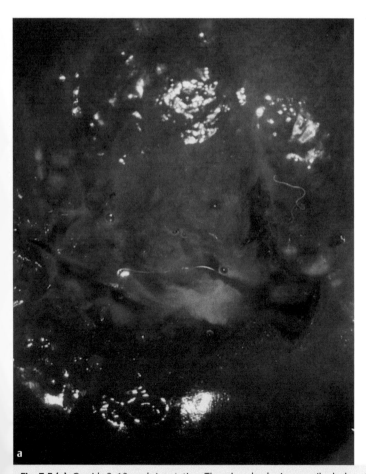

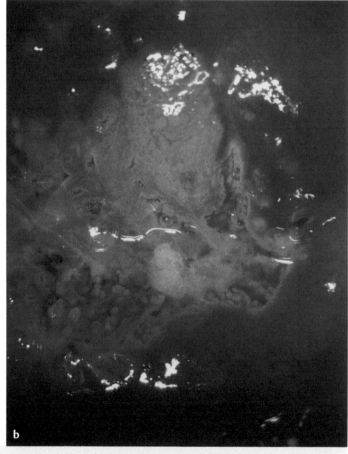

Fig. 7.5 (a) Gravida 2, 18 weeks' gestation. There is a clearly circumscribed, almost unstructured area within an otherwise unremarkable transformation zone on the anterior lip. **(b)** After application of acetic acid, a few gland openings and a fine mosaic appear within the area described. Histology showed metaplastic epithelium.

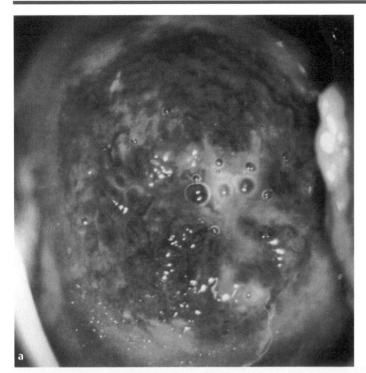 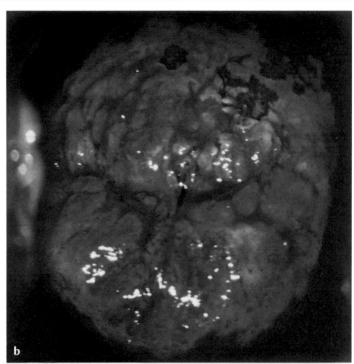

Fig. 7.6 (a) Gravida 2, 11 weeks' gestation. Preexistent transformation zone (TZ) with a slightly coarse surface and increased vascularity. Slightly livid coloration of the original cervical epithelium. **(b)** After application of iodine (Schiller's test), the squamous epithelium is stained dark brown. Within the TZ, there are islands of a mature, glycogen-containing metaplastic epithelium.

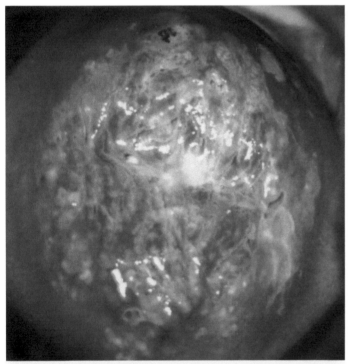 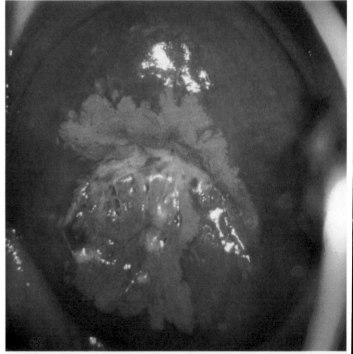

Fig. 7.7 Gravida 1, 8 weeks' gestation. Transformation zone, with a whitish reaction to acetic acid. Cuffed gland openings. Flat condylomas between 12 o'clock and 2 o'clock positions.

Fig. 7.8 Gravida 1, 11 weeks' gestation. After acetic acid, a white area with fine mosaic and punctation appears on the anterior and posterior lip inside the transformation zone. The border with the slightly livid original epithelium is sharp. Histology showed metaplastic epithelium.

toward contact bleeding are observed with introduction of the speculum, especially when taking a smear or biopsy.

The lividity and softness bring about background changes in the colposcopic appearance. In contrast to the nonpregnant state, these are coarse and may give even benign changes a suspicious and alarming aspect (Figs. 7.5–7.9). This applies especially to the response to acetic acid.

7.1.1 Acetic Acid Test

The effect of acetic acid is more pronounced during pregnancy, so that whitening even of benign lesions can appear suspicious (Figs. 7.5b, 7.7, and 7.9b). Thus, the response to acetic acid can be difficult to interpret during pregnancy.

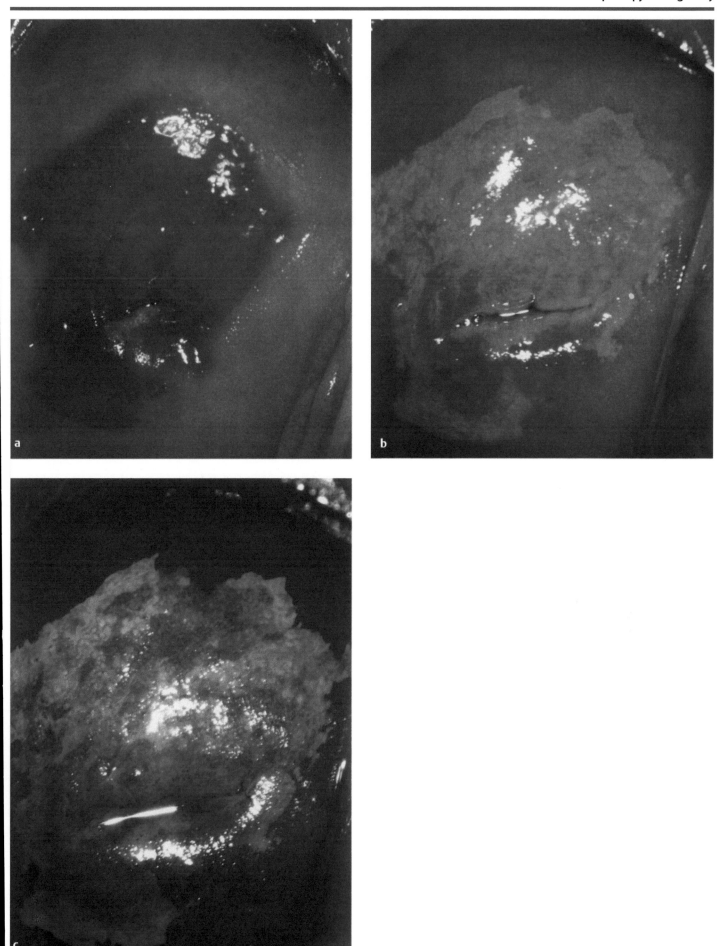

Fig. 7.9 (a) Gravida 1, 11 weeks' gestation. Shiny red area within the livid squamous epithelium. **(b)** After acetic acid, the entire area turns white, but without swelling. There are small areas of fine mosaic. An isolated field can be delineated between the 11 o'clock and 12 o'clock positions. **(c)** After application of iodine, there is a patchy, partly brown staining of the previously completely white area. Histology showed metaplastic epithelium.

7.1.2 Schiller's (Iodine) Test

The Schiller's test is affected by pregnancy only to the extent that the cervicovaginal squamous epithelium turns a more intense brownish black with iodine (Figs. 7.6b, 7.10, and 7.11b). The Schiller's test is particularly useful when an area that turns white after acetic acid displays a speckled, but not uniform, brown appearance with iodine (Fig. 7.9c). Such a finding suggests a condylomatous lesion rather than atypia.

Postpartum, especially in breastfeeding mothers, colposcopy can show areas on the cervix and vagina that do not stain with iodine. This epithelium is glycogen-free as a result of postpartum atrophy (Fig. 7.12b). After cessation of breastfeeding, conditions revert to normal, with the usual uniform staining of the vagina and cervix.

7.2 Benign Changes in Pregnancy

At the beginning of pregnancy, the cervix is largely unchanged (Fig. 7.13) and shows the coarse, grapelike appearance of ectopy. The longitudinal folds of the cervical mucosa are particularly distinctive (Fig. 7.4). Such appearances can be elicited merely by everting the endocervical canal with the speculum. The coarsening of the surface contour of the transformation zone (TZ) can occur early in pregnancy (Fig. 7.6a). The Schiller's test can bring out other diagnostic features, including islands of mature, glycogen-rich epithelium. The indistinct border between the TZ and the surrounding iodine-positive cervix is also suggestive of a benign lesion (Fig. 7.6b). After

acetic acid is applied, a normal TZ often turns more intensely acetowhite than usual, with more prominent gland openings (Figs. 7.7 and 7.14). When transformation is complete, one can see retention cysts and gland openings shining through the lucid epithelium (Fig. 7.4).

Clearly delineated areas within a normal TZ can appear suspicious, especially when they display an intense and prompt reaction to acetic acid (Fig. 7.5a, b). In pregnancy, this applies especially to metaplastic epithelium, which can also be clearly demarcated from original squamous epithelium and can show mosaic, punctation, or both (Fig. 7.8). In such cases, the small size and regular appearance of the mosaic, or delicate and regular punctation, provide helpful diagnostic hints. In the case of some coarser-looking lesions, and certain combinations of changes, it may be difficult or impossible to make an exact colposcopic diagnosis (Fig. 7.9a–c).

The decidual reaction can barely be seen colposcopically, as it manifests itself in the deeper cervical stroma. Decidual polyps, however, are easily distinguished from conventional endocervical polyps. The latter often are covered by smooth, pink metaplastic squamous epithelium (Fig. 6.108) or display the typical grapelike pattern of columnar epithelium, whereas decidual polyps are yellowish and not covered by epithelium (Figs. 7.1–7.3).

Condylomatous lesions are relatively common in pregnancy. Except for a certain softness, they are similar to those in the nonpregnant patient (Fig. 7.15). Inflammatory lesions look the same as they do outside pregnancy. Because the normal squamous epithelium has a deeper brown color, they stand out strongly after iodine (Fig. 7.10; see also Fig. 6.103b).

7.3 Suspicious Changes

Colposcopic findings corresponding to SIL (CIN) are rather uniform in pregnancy. The distinction between LSIL and metaplastic epithelium is difficult (Figs. 7.5, 7.8, 7.9, and 7.16). An irregular, coarser appearance of mosaic, for example, suggests HSIL (as it does outside of pregnancy). Lesions can occur just outside the TZ (Figs. 7.11 and 7.17). Lividity can give an abnormal colposcopic finding a particular hue (Fig. 7.18), which can be overlooked or interpreted as harmless. In other cases, one may find an abnormal appearance with strong white coloration of the sharply circumscribed TZ (Fig. 7.19). Bright red lesions are particularly striking, are always suspicious, and, in cases of HSIL, also respond characteristically to acetic acid (Fig. 7.20a, b).

Condylomas can lose their typical pearly-white appearance (Fig. 6.98) during pregnancy. They can assume a dark red undertone, which makes them difficult to recognize as condylomas (Fig. 7.21a). An important diagnostic aid in such cases is the application of iodine (Schiller's test), which elicits a distinctive brown staining, with sparing of small clear patches, producing a speckled appearance (Fig. 7.21b). This appearance corresponds to the iodine-positive mosaic in Fig. 6.98b. During the course of the pregnancy, it can become coarser, more livid, and more succulent (Fig. 7.21c, d). After the puerperium, one can often observe the regression of condylomas (Fig. 7.21e), which merely displays islands of brown-staining epithelium at the periphery (Fig. 7.21f).

7.4 The Puerperium

Lesions established during pregnancy remain essentially unchanged during the puerperium but lose the characteristic features of pregnancy (Figs. 7.12a and 7.21a–f). The Schiller's test can reveal surprising findings: parts of the cervix and varying lengths of the corrugated surface of the vagina remain unstained (i.e., glycogen-free) (Fig. 7.12a, b), particularly in breastfeeding women. The appearances are probably caused by the hypoestrogenic state induced by lactation and revert to normal after cessation of lactation.

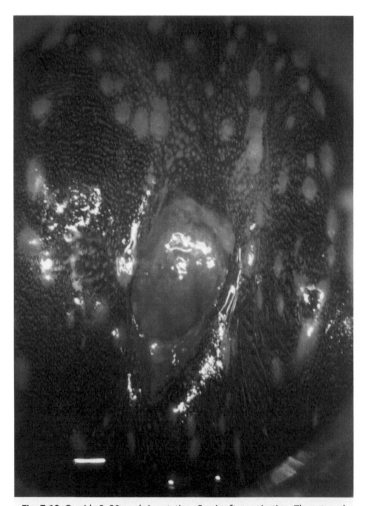

Fig. 7.10 Gravida 8, 20 weeks' gestation. Cervix after conization. The external os is slit-like; the mucosa on the anterior lip is slightly everted. The plaques of macular colpitis are distinct from the dark brown cervical squamous epithelium.

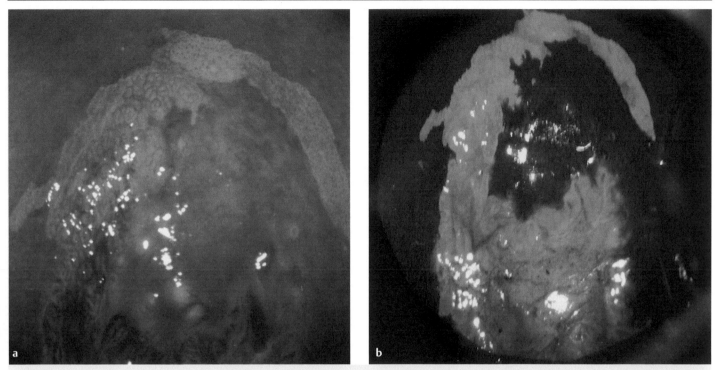

Fig. 7.11 (a) Gravida 2. A livid transformation zone (TZ) on the anterior lip, with mature metaplastic squamous epithelium and retention cysts shining through. The TZ is semicircularly surrounded by a narrow band of fairly coarse, irregular mosaic. Histology showed HSIL (CIN 2). **(b)** At a lower magnification, and after application of iodine (Schiller's test), the narrow band with the mosaic is sharply demarcated. The epithelium in the completed TZ on the anterior lip is stained dark brown. On the posterior lip, there is an early TZ with a diffuse border.

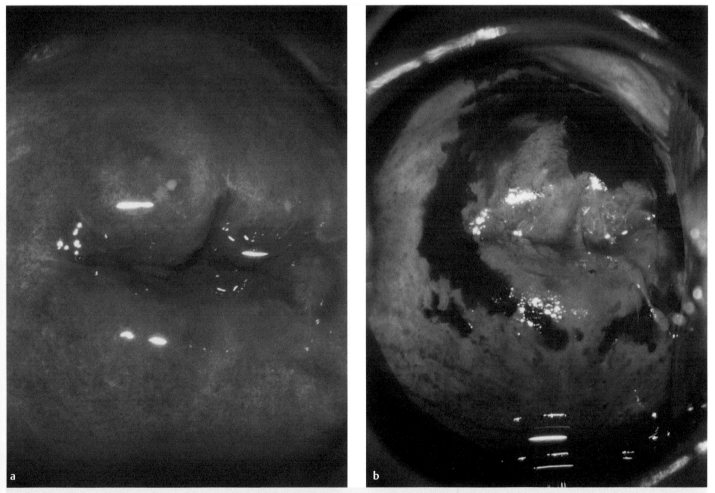

Fig. 7.12 (a) Four weeks after delivery. The cervix is still slightly red and edematous, with a narrow transformation zone. **(b)** After the Schiller's test, surprisingly large areas of the cervix and vagina are not stained (i.e., glycogen-free). Islands of brown staining appear within these areas.

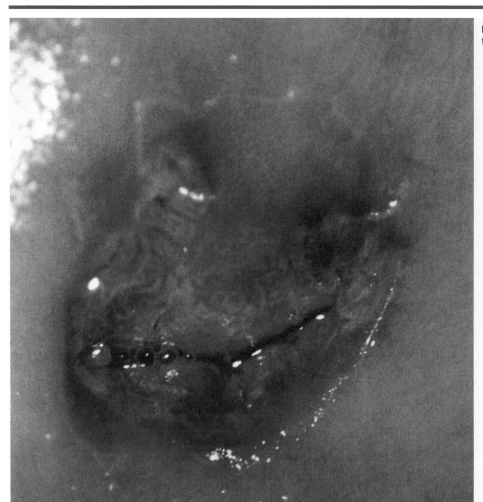

Fig. 7.13 Gravida 5, 10 weeks' gestation. Narrow transformation zone, slight lividity.

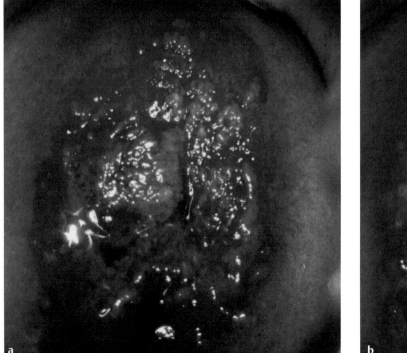

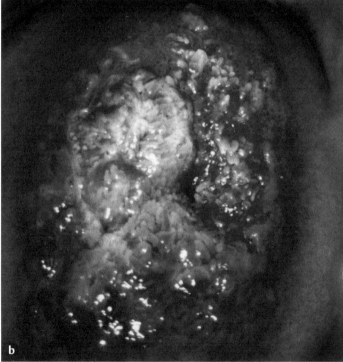

Fig. 7.14 (a) Gravida 2, 13 weeks' gestation. Ectopy and transformation zone (TZ) with elevated decidual foci on the posterior lip of the cervix. **(b)** After application of 3% acetic acid, the columnar epithelium swells markedly but the TZ and the decidual foci remain largely unchanged.

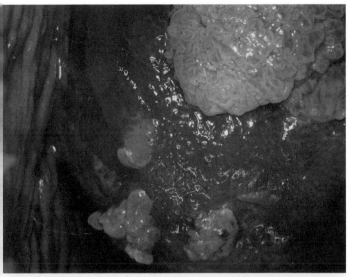

Fig. 7.15 Thirty weeks' gestation. Papillary condylomas, around the external os. The vagina and cervix are highly congested. Within this lesion and at its edge are condylomatous excrescences that have also assumed a deep red color.

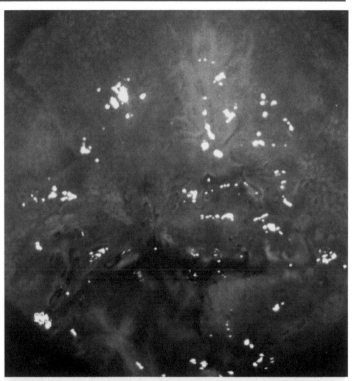

Fig. 7.16 Gravida 1, 20 weeks' gestation. Acetic acid has been applied. Outside the transformation zone, on the anterior lip of the external os, there is a fairly fine mosaic, sharply demarcated from its surroundings. Histology showed LSIL (CIN 1).

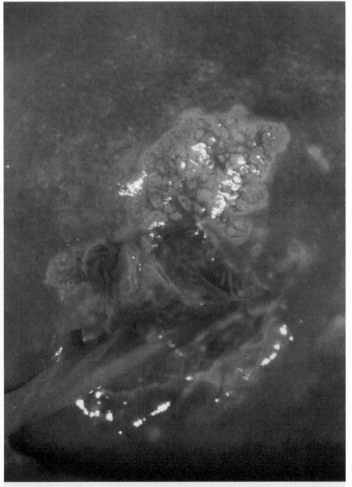

Fig. 7.17 Gravida 1, 16 weeks' gestation. After application of acetic acid, an irregular, coarse mosaic appears at the edge of the ectopy and outside the transformation zone. Histology showed HSIL (CIN 2).

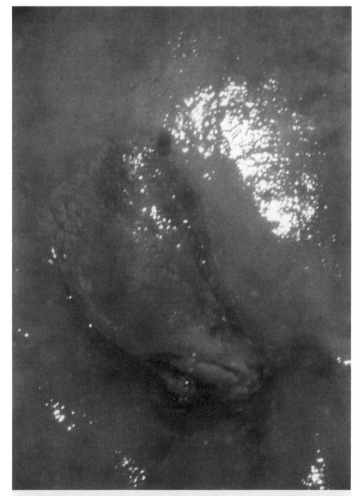

Fig. 7.18 Gravida 2, 10 weeks' gestation. After application of acetic acid, a deeply livid tongue-like area appears on the posterior lip. Within this area are only isolated gland openings; at its edge, there is a narrow band with coarse mosaic. Histology showed HSIL (CIN 2).

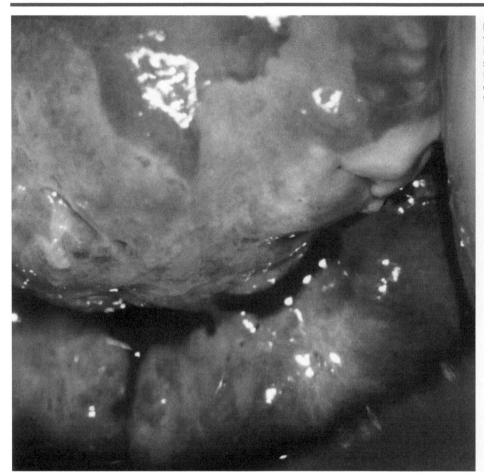

Fig. 7.19 Gravida 4, 40 weeks' gestation. The transformation zone with isolated gland openings is stained intensely white by acetic acid and is sharply demarcated. Ridge sign at 4 o'clock position. Histology showed HSIL (CIN 3), which was followed closely over the pregnancy. The bleeding resulted from a smear taken with an Ayre's spatula.

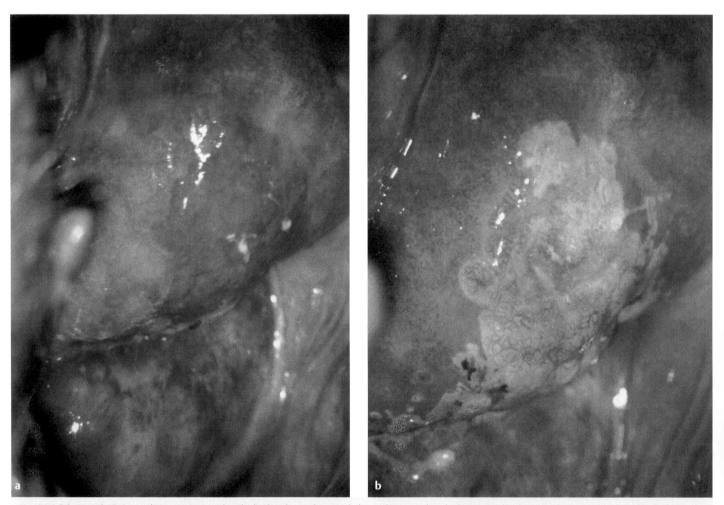

Fig. 7.20 (a) Gravida 7, 29 weeks' gestation. Within the livid and succulent epithelium, there is a sharply demarcated red area without any recognizable surface structure. **(b)** After application of acetic acid, the area swells, and a coarse mosaic appears. Histology showed HSIL (CIN 3).

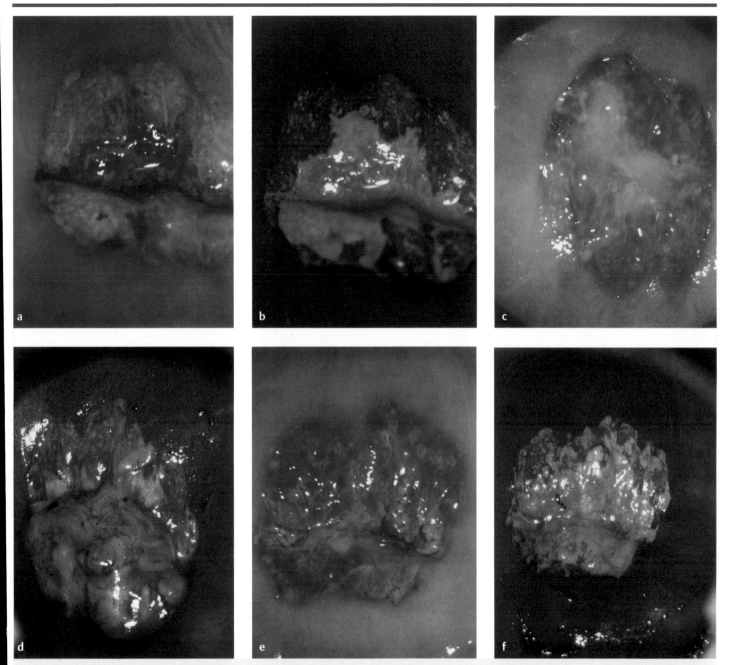

Fig. 7.21 (a) Gravida 2, 8 weeks' gestation. At the edge of an ectopy undergoing transformation, there is white-to-livid epithelium with cervical gland openings and white dots. The dots correspond to crypt involvement of squamous epithelium. Histology showed HSIL (CIN 2) with koilocytosis. **(b)** Brown staining after application of iodine confirms a flat condyloma (LSIL). The small, light spots could be called iodine-positive punctation. **(c)** By 24 weeks' gestation, the lesion has become coarser and succulent. **(d)** With the Schiller's test, the staining of the epithelium on the anterior lip is unchanged. Mucus prevents staining of the posterior lip. **(e)** Six weeks after delivery, the transformation zone (TZ) appears normal and bright red. The lesion has become smaller. Histology showed metaplastic squamous epithelium. **(f)** Application of iodine produces only patchy staining at the edge of the TZ.

7.5 Biopsy during Pregnancy

Colposcopy in pregnancy is used to rule out invasive cervical cancer. It is quite possible to perform a punch biopsy of the cervix during pregnancy. Bleeding can be controlled with a tampon, which should be left in for a few hours. Careful endocervical curettage can also be performed when indicated; naturally, this should not reach the upper confines of the endocervical canal, where lesions are rare during pregnancy.

Further Reading

Ahdoot D, Van Nostrand KM, Nguyen NJ, et al. The effect of route of delivery on regression of abnormal cervical cytologic findings in the postpartum period. Am J Obstet Gynecol 1998;178:1116–1120

Fader AN, Alward EK, Niederhauser A, et al. Cervical dysplasia in pregnancy: a multi-institutional evaluation. Am J Obstet Gynecol 2010;203:113.e1–113.e6

Fitzgerald PJ, Marsh M. Carcinoma in situ of the human uterine cervix in pregnancy; prevalence and postpregnancy persistence. Cancer 1956;9: 1195–1207

Fleury AC, Birsner ML, Fader AN. Management of the abnormal Papanicolaou smear and colposcopy in pregnancy: an evidenced-based review. Minerva Ginecol 2012;64: 137–148

Freeman-Wang T, Walker P. Colposcopy in special circumstances: pregnancy, immunocompromise, adolescence and menopause. Best Pract Res Clin Obstet Gynaecol 2011;25:653–665

Mailath-Pokorny M, Schwameis R, Grimm C, Reinthaller A, Polterauer S. Natural history of cervical intraepithelial neoplasia in pregnancy: postpartum histo-pathologic outcome and review of the literature. BMC Pregnancy Childbirth 2016;16:74

Morice P, Uzan C, Gouy S, Verschraegen C, Haie-Meder C. Gynecological cancers in pregnancy. Lancet 2012;379(9815):558–569

Trutnovsky G, Kolovetsiou-Kreiner V, Reich O. p16/Ki-67 dual-stained cytology testing may predict postpartum outcome in patients with abnormal papanicolaou cytology during pregnancy. Acta Cytol 2014;58:293–296

Wetta LA, Matthews KS, Kemper ML, et al. The management of cervical intraepithelial neoplasia during pregnancy: is colposcopy necessary? J Low Genit Tract Dis 2009;13:182–185

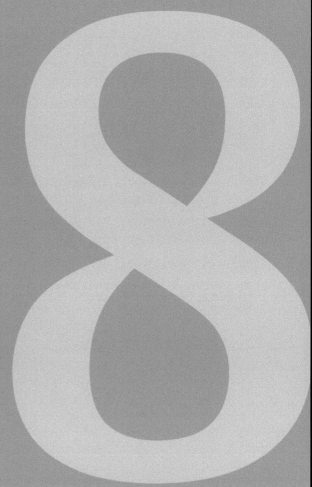

Chapter 8

Colposcopy of the Vulva

8 Colposcopy of the Vulva

8.1 Histology of the Vulva

The vulva is covered by three types of squamous epithelium:
- **Keratinized skin** with hair follicles, sebaceous glands, and apocrine and eccrine sweat glands. This type of skin covers the mons pubis and the labia majora.
- **Modified mucosa** with sebaceous glands but no hair follicles or sweat glands; no cornification on the interlabial sulci covers the outer aspect of the labia minora and the clitoris.
- **Glycogen-containing mucosa** without sebaceous or sweat glands, hair, or cornification covers the inner aspect of the labia minora and the introitus (Fig. 8.1).

The transition between the keratinized and nonkeratinized epithelia (Hart's line) is sometimes visible to the naked eye and always visible microscopically. Hart's line is best seen at the posterior fourchette, and it marks the peripheral border of the vaginal vestibulum. The vaginal vestibulum comprises the outer aspect of the hymen, which separates the vestibule from the vagina, the frenulum clitoridis, the inner aspect of the labia minora, the vaginal introitus, and the external urethral orifice.

The epidermis is a stratified squamous epithelium composed of distinct layers. In a vertical section, the epidermis has an undulating appearance caused by the malpighian rete. The deepest layer, resting on the basement membrane, is the basal cell layer (germinative layer, stratum germinativum) from which the epithelium regenerates. The basal cells are undifferentiated and pluripotent. The basal layer also contains melanocytes, which are highly differentiated. The spinal cell layer (stratum spinosum) is the layer most variable in thickness. The next layer, the granular layer (stratum granulosum), is followed by the horny layer (stratum corneum), which also varies in thickness.

A variant of normal is the so-called *micropapillomatosis*. These are prominent, 1- to 3-mm vestibular papillae (Fig. 8.2), which are a common finding in premenopausal women and are not to be confused with condylomas. Micropapillomatosis can also be found at the inner aspect of the labia minora and at the external edges of the vestibule.

The glycogen-containing mucosa of the introitus and the vagina has the same appearance as the cervical epithelium and is very sensitive to hormonal influences. With lack of estrogen in childhood and after menopause, this layer is thin. With exposure to estrogen, the mucosa gains its characteristic multilayered appearance. Apart from the basal cell layer, which does not contain melanocytes, the next cell layers are generally uniform. All contain glycogen in the cytoplasm, which gives it a honeycomb appearance in hematoxylin–eosin sections. Apart from the basal cell layer, one can distinguish only an intermediate and a superficial cell layer.

The vulva can be affected nonspecifically by dermatologic conditions and by specific conditions. The vulva is an epithelial high-risk area with a predisposition to multifocal and recurrent malignant transformation.

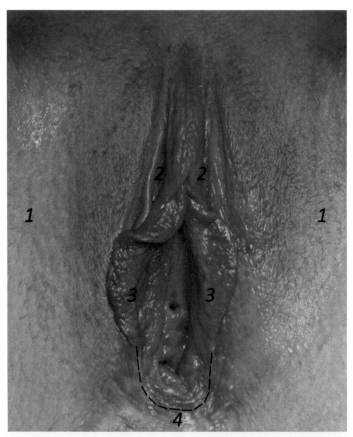

Fig. 8.1 Three types of vulvar squamous epithelium: **1** Keratinized skin; **2** modified mucosa; and **3** glycogen-containing mucosa. Hart's line (**4**) is the border between the keratinized and nonkeratinized epithelia.

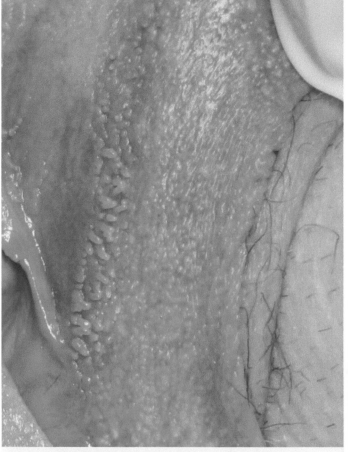

Fig. 8.2 Micropapillomatosis at the inner aspect of the labia minora.

8.2 Diagnostic Methods for Evaluating Vulvar Lesions

The diagnosis of vulvar disorders is based on the clinical history, inspection, palpation, colposcopy, histology, and, in some instances, confirmation with laboratory evaluation, including biomarkers.

8.2.1 History and Symptoms

In younger patients, the history is often brief and related to an acute condition. Older patients frequently have chronic lesions, and sometimes there is a marked discrepancy between the subjective complaints and the objective findings. Characteristic symptoms of vulvar lesions are itching (pruritus), soreness, burning sensations, paresthesias, and pain, including dyspareunia. The relevant surgical, medical (diabetes), and psychiatric history should be elicited. Medications, estrogen replacement, allergies, incontinence, and prior vaginitis and sexually transmitted diseases are of interest.

8.2.2 Inspection

Diseases of the vulva vary and overlap in appearance. Some patients have multiple conditions. Biopsy and histopathology are required for most diagnoses. Vulvar lesions that do not resolve within weeks of medical management have to be watched closely to detect progression. Photographic documentation is very helpful (Table 8.1).

8.2.3 Palpation

Many vulvar conditions are normal to palpation. However, even small invasive carcinomas show a tougher consistency around their base than the surrounding tissue. Small invasive foci may, on occasion, be suspected in large areas of abnormal findings by palpation alone. When these lesions grow, they are no longer at the level of the surrounding tissue and become less mobile against the dermis. The surface of vulvar conditions can also be smooth or rough on palpation; a rough surface is often due to either crust or scale.

8.2.4 Toluidine Blue Test (Collins' Test)

This technique, now rarely used, consists of 1% toluidine blue dye applied to the vulva for 2 to 3 minutes and then washed off with 1% acetic acid (Fig. 8.3). The toluidine blue test can also be used during surgery to plan the margins of the excision. However, the test has become almost obsolete with the increased use of colposcopy with acetic acid. Colposcopy (vulvoscopy) provides much more detail, particularly for papillary lesions and the typical findings of punctations and mosaics. Toluidine blue is sometimes applied for forensic purposes to demonstrate injuries.

8.2.5 Colposcopy of the Vulva

Magnification of the vulvar skin with or without the application of acetic acid permits more precise evaluation and earlier detection of vulvar lesions than inspection with the naked eye. In contrast to colposcopy of the cervix, low magnification usually suffices.

Color can be described as red (erythroplakia), white (leukoplakia), or pigmented (melanotic). Skin-colored lesions are those that match the color of the surrounding normal skin. In the mucosal portion of the vulva, skin-colored lesions will be pink or red. Evaluation of color does not require colposcopy.

Redness (*erythroplakia*) can be due to acute or chronic inflammation, squamous intraepithelial lesions (SIL), differentiated-type vulvar intraepithelial neoplasia (dVIN), or invasive neoplasia. Erythroplakia can be circumscribed or diffuse (Figs. 8.4 and 8.5).

Leukoplakia is a general descriptive term for whitish lesions before application of acetic acid. It is caused by thickening of the superficial keratinized epithelial layers. Whiteness can be caused by dermatoses such as lichen sclerosus or lichen planus with decreased blood supply and hyperkeratosis as well as with malignant and premalignant conditions (Figs. 8.6–8.8).

Dark (melanotic) lesions: Apart from the lesions of malignant melanoma and its precursors, about 30% of all high-grade SIL (HSIL) are associated with irregular hyperpigmentation (Fig. 8.9).

Colposcopy of the vulva is used for the following:
- To define the extent of lesions.
- To direct biopsies to the area of the most clinically severe abnormality.
- To exclude overt invasive cancer.
- To direct treatment by visualizing anatomic landmarks.

The 2011 IFCPC Clinical/Colposcopic Terminology of the Vulva distinguishes normal findings, abnormal findings, miscellaneous findings, findings suspicious for malignancy, and abnormal colposcopic (magnification) findings. *Sharp borders* are also important. *Mosaic* is not included in the new terminology, although it can be detected in vulvar lesions. The vulvar terminology does not distinguish between minor and major abnormal colposcopic findings, as it does for the cervix and vagina.

Acetowhite epithelium. In contrast to the cervix, where acetic acid is an integral part of the examination, on the vulva, acetic acid is applied only when morphologic manifestation of HPV

Table 8.1 Secondary morphology presentation

Type of lesion	Comment
Eczema	A group of inflammatory diseases that are clinically characterized by the presence of itchy, poorly marginated red plaques with minor evidence of microvesiculation and/or, more frequently, subsequent surface disruption
Lichenification	Thickening of the tissue and increased prominence of skin markings. Scale may or may not be detectable in vulvar lichenification. Lichenification may be bright red, dusky red, white, or skin-colored
Excoriation	Surface disruption occurring as a result of the "itch–scratch cycle"
Erosion	A shallow defect in the skin surface; absence of some, or all, of the epidermis down to the basement membrane; the dermis is intact
Fissure	A thin, linear erosion of the skin surface
Ulcer	Deeper defect; absence of the epidermis and some, or all, of the dermis

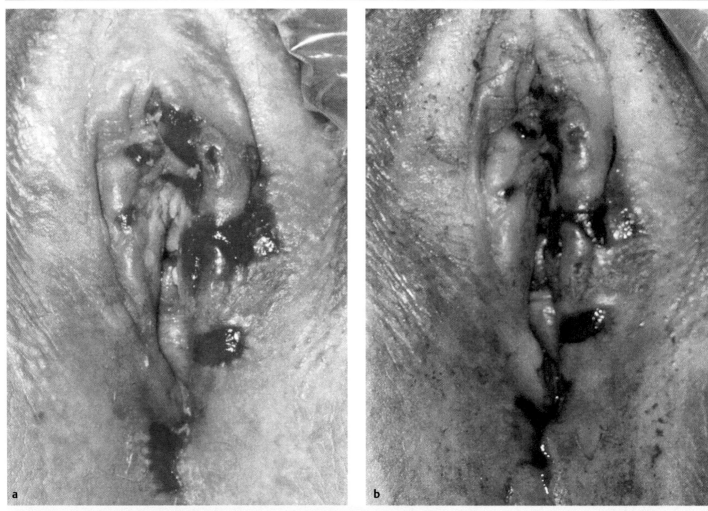

Fig. 8.3 Collins' test. **(a)** Multicentric erosions in a patient with lichen sclerosus. **(b)** Positive toluidine blue staining of the erosions. The test is unspecific because staining is seen with both dysplastic and neoplastic lesions as well as benign injuries, erosions, and ulcers.

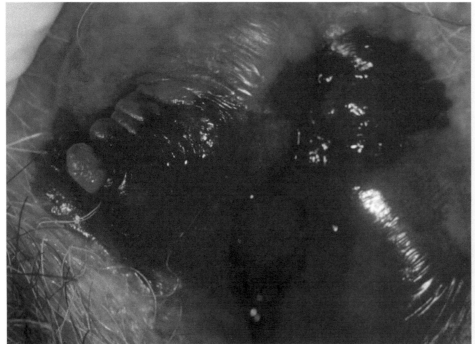

Fig. 8.4 Erythroplakia in a patient with HSIL.

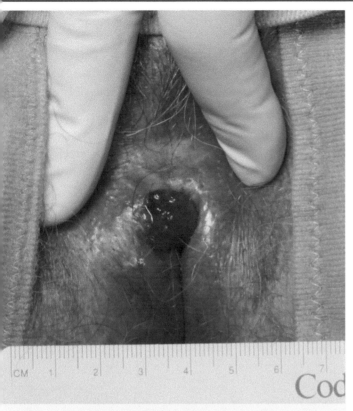

Fig. 8.5 Erythroplakia in a patient with small HPV-associated invasive vulvar cancer.

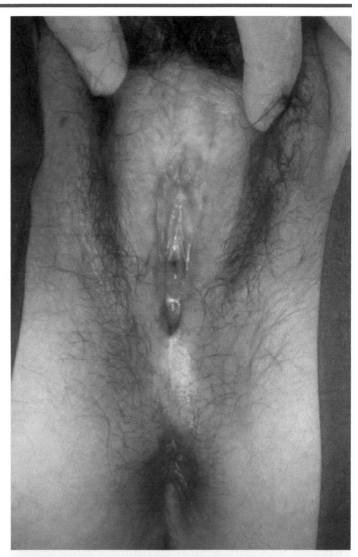

Fig. 8.6 Leukoplakia in a patient with advanced lichen sclerosus.

infection (SIL) or early invasive disease linked to high-risk HPV is suspected. Application of 3 to 5% acetic acid requires 2 to 3 minutes for lesions to become apparent.

It is important to carefully inspect the vulva before acetic acid is applied in order to outline preexisting areas of leukoplakia. Diffuse and flat acetowhite epithelium can represent a normal finding that is most likely due to increased cell turnover secondary to mechanical stimuli or inflammatory conditions of the vulva. Flat acetowhite epithelium therefore should be considered nonspecific. In contrast, acetowhite epithelium from HSIL is more likely to be raised and sharply demarcated. The results after application of acetic acid are interpreted in combination with other signs such as punctation, mosaic, sharp borders, elevated lesions, and atypical vessels (Fig. 8.10).

Punctation and mosaic. Acetowhite epithelium, erythroplakia, and leukoplakia can show *mosaics* and *punctations* when studied with the colposcope. They are more common in the nonkeratinizing, glycogen-containing squamous epithelium of the introitus than in the remaining vulva (Figs. 8.11–8.14).

Sharp borders. Border zones (margination) represent the transition from normal skin to lesional skin. A sharply marginated lesion has an abrupt transition; a poorly marginated lesion has a more gradual transition. HSIL are often sharply demarcated from their surrounding normal epithelium, as are different types of abnormal epithelia among themselves (Fig. 8.15). The larger the difference in the differentiation of areas of adjoining HSIL, the clearer the border between them. In contrast, inflammation affects the stroma more than the epithelium and its borders are much less defined. Sharp demarcation is seen with carcinomas of all sizes (Fig. 8.16).

Surface irregularities. Leukoplakias with a rough and irregular surface are suspicious for dVIN (see section 8.3.2).

Atypical vessels. As at other locations, atypical vessels are suggestive of invasive lesions (Fig. 8.17).

The 2011 IFCPC terminology for the vulva distinguishes primary lesion types (Table 7.5) and secondary presentations (Table 8.1). These lesions can be evaluated with the naked eye, a magnifying glass, or a colposcope with low magnification.

8.2.6 Assessment of Colposcopic Findings

Acetowhite epithelium. Sharply demarcated and raised acetowhite epithelium generally corresponds to HSIL, whereas dVIN generally does not react to acetic acid.

Leukoplakia and erythroplakia. SIL and dVIN can cause marked hyper/parakeratosis visible as leukoplakia or inflammation and hypervascularization visible as erythroplakia. There are also erythroplakic areas in atrophic glycogen-containing squamous epithelium.

Punctation and mosaic. Punctations and mosaics in nonmalignant lesions correspond to thin epithelial ridges and wide stromal papillae. In premalignant and malignant lesions, the stromal papillae are much narrower and the epithelial ridges plumper and more irregular. In vertical sections, the differences between normal and atypical squamous epithelium are even more apparent. Papillae and papillary ridges of considerable height can be seen in hyperplastic epidermis as well as in all types of SIL. High and thin stromal papillae in papillary low-grade SIL (LSIL) are especially well seen. Papillomatous HSIL often show marked but irregular stromal papillae.

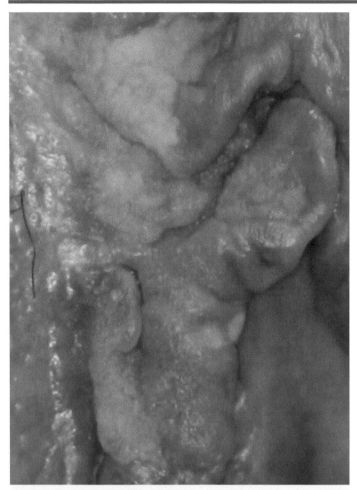

Fig. 8.7 Leukoplakia in a patient with multicentric HSIL.

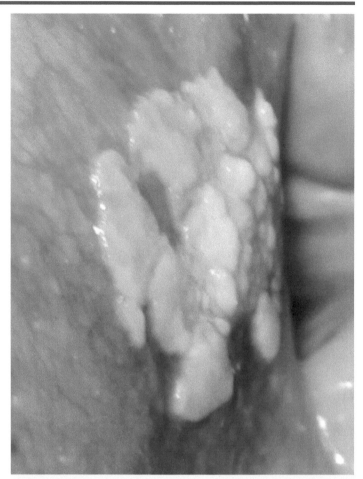

Fig. 8.8 Leukoplakia, well circumscribed, at the introitus vaginae. Histology shows HSIL.

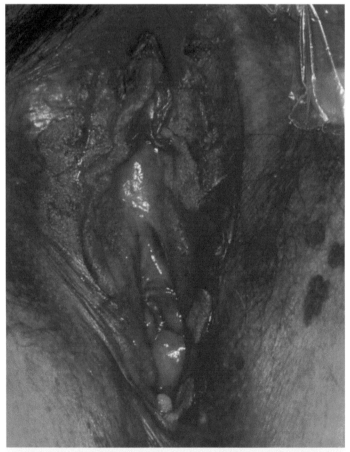

Fig. 8.9 Irregular hyperpigmentation in a patient with multicentric HSIL.

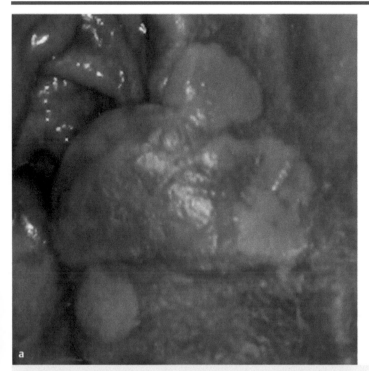
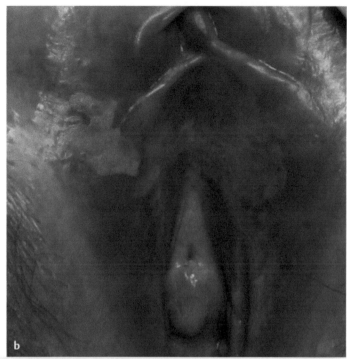

Fig. 8.10 Acetowhite epithelium **(a)** raised in a patient with HSIL **(b)** sharply demarcated. Histology showed HSIL.

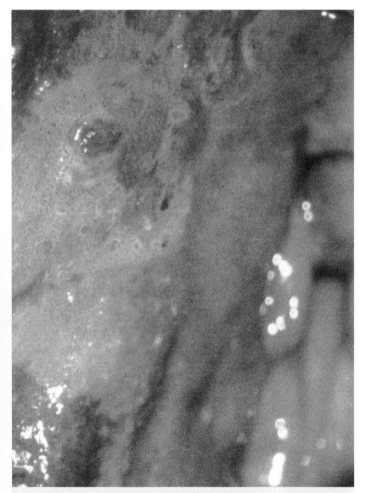

Fig. 8.11 Acetowhite epithelium with marked punctation and a slight mosaic in a patient with HSIL.

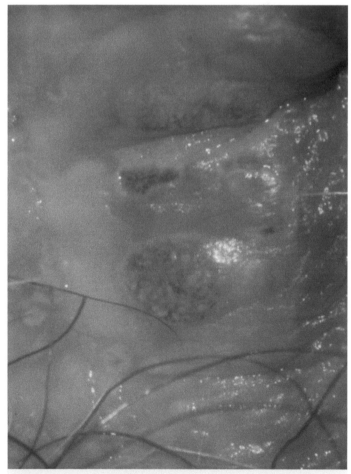

Fig. 8.12 Coarse mosaic with sharp borders surrounded by acetowhite epithelium in a patient with FIGO I HPV 16–positive vulvar squamous cell carcinoma.

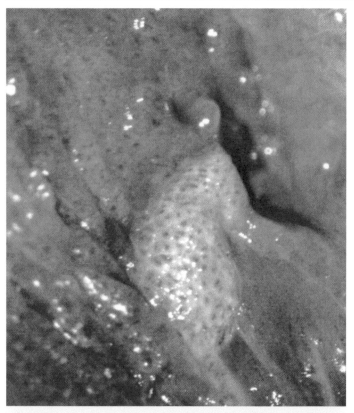

Fig. 8.13 Coarse punctation in an elevated acetowhite epithelium. Histology shows HSIL.

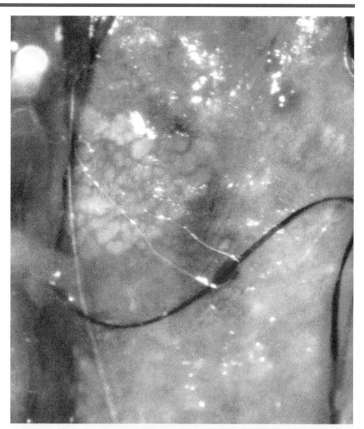

Fig. 8.14 Coarse mosaic in a lesion with leukoplakia. Histology shows HSIL.

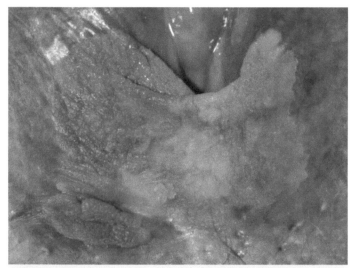

Fig. 8.15 Sharp borders in a slightly pigmented lesion with rough leukoplakia and surface irregularities. Histology showed HSIL.

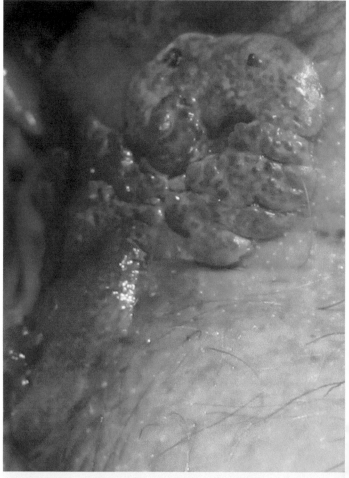

Fig. 8.16 Sharp borders of a FIGO stage I HPV 16–positive squamous cell vulvar cancer.

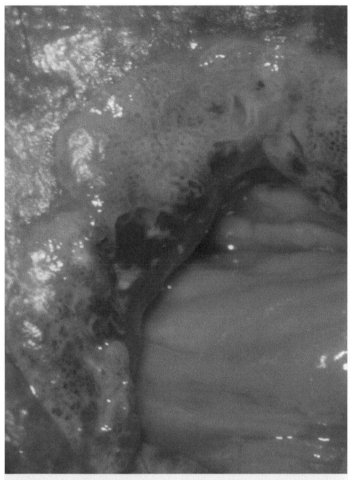

Fig. 8.17 Fragile atypical vessels in an exophytic, well-demarcated FIGO stage II squamous cell vulvar cancer.

8.2.7 Biopsy

Biopsy should be performed on all suspicious lesions of the vulva, including white, gray, red, pigmented, or raised lesions and all conditions that do not resolve promptly with medical treatment. If the lesion is uniform, a single biopsy suffices. If the lesion is multifaceted, two or more biopsies should be obtained. In ulcerative lesions, a biopsy at the periphery can avoid nonrepresentative necrosis.

Biopsies can be performed quickly and simply with local anesthesia (lidocaine with or without adrenaline or topical lidocaine cream) on an outpatient basis using just a few instruments (Fig. 8.18). The hands of the patient can help expose the lesion. A 5-mm punch biopsy perpendicular to the surface is ideal. The defect on occasion requires a fine resorbable suture for hemostasis. Ideally, anticoagulants are discontinued before biopsy.

8.2.8 Exfoliative Cytology

Cytology has poor sensitivity and specificity for the detection of SIL. Liquid-based cytology may provide better results than conventional cytology, especially at the mucosal side of the vulva. Cytology is inadequate in the detection of dVIN, Paget's disease, and melanoma in situ.

8.2.9 HPV Testing

HPV testing permits differentiation between low-risk and high-risk infections as well as between (pre)neoplastic conditions associated with HPV and lesions not associated with HPV. HPV testing is also important to define the risk of progression in LSIL because LSIL containing low-risk

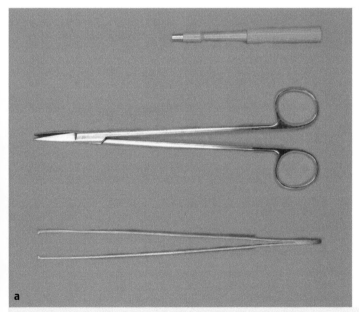

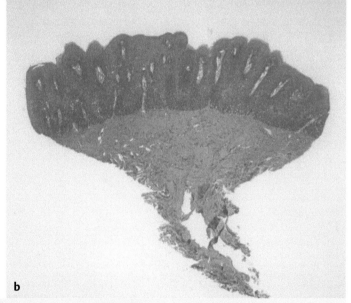

Fig. 8.18 Punch biopsy. **(a)** Required instruments. **(b)** The biopsy specimen contains epithelium and underlying stroma.

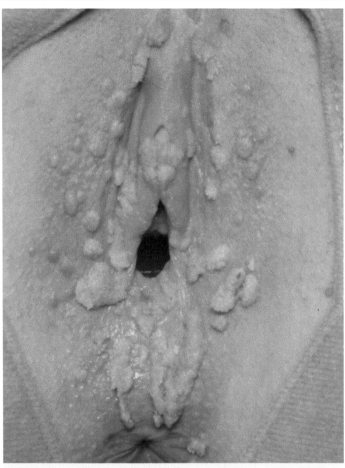

Fig. 8.19 Condyloma acuminata.

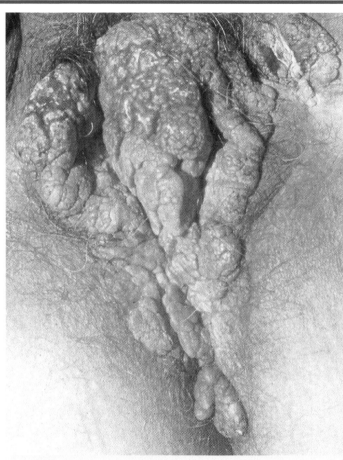

Fig. 8.20 Giant condyloma (Buschke–Löwenstein) with malignant transformation. These tumors are due to low-risk HPV types.

Table 8.2 Characteristics of the two types of squamous cell carcinoma (SCC) of the vulva

	HPV-associated SCC	HPV-negative SCC
Etiology	Transforming HPV infection, predominantly HPV 16	Long-standing lichen sclerosus or lichen planus
Frequency	40%	60%
Age at diagnosis	Younger	Older
Precursor lesions	SIL	dVIN
Possible molecular pathogenesis	High-risk HPV infection; viral E6/E7 expression, inactivation of p53 and retinoblastoma gene, genetic instability, DNA aneuploidy	Immunodysregulation, mutation of p53/PTEN, allelic imbalance, microsatellite instability, DNA aneuploidy
Progression time	Slower	Faster
Prognosis	Better (?)	Worse (?)
Prevention	HPV vaccination	Treatment of underlying dermatosis (?)

Abbreviations: HPV, human papillomavirus; PTEN, phosphatase and tensin homolog; dVIN, vulvar intraepithelial neoplasia, differentiated type.

HPV is histologically indistinguishable from LSIL containing high-risk HPV. HPV testing has a role in the follow-up of patients after treatment for HPV-positive lesions (Figs. 8.19 and 8.20).

8.3 Vulvar Carcinogenesis

Two distinct pathways, one HPV-associated and one HPV-independent, are involved in vulvar carcinogenesis (Table 8.2). Typically, HPV-associated carcinogenesis results in warty or basaloid-type squamous cell carcinoma (SCC) via SIL (Fig. 8.21),

whereas HPV-independent carcinogenesis results in keratinizing-type SCC, via dVIN. However, there is some overlap between the histologic types and the association with HPV. Some HPV-positive vulvar SCCs are keratinizing, and a few HPV-negative vulvar SCCs show basaloid or warty features.

Vulvar cancers develop over a variable period of time. Typically, HPV-associated vulvar SCCs occur in relatively young women, whereas HPV-negative cancers are commonly found in older patients. Although HPV-associated SCCs of the head and neck region have a better prognosis than HPV-independent SCCs, it is unclear whether this is true for vulvar cancers.

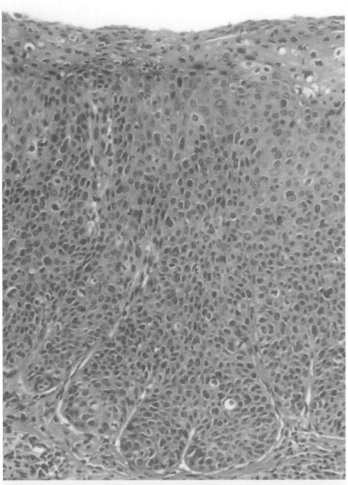

Fig. 8.21 Basaloid SIL with a flat surface. This variant of SIL has smaller cells with less cellular pleomorphism than warty VIN.

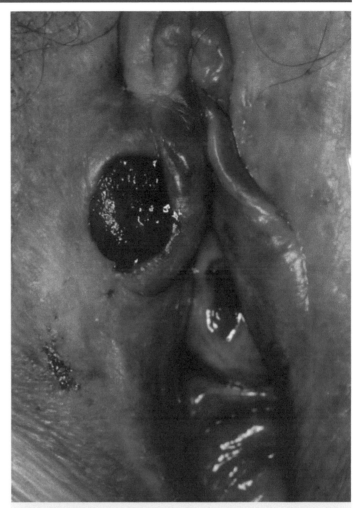

Fig. 8.22 HPV 16–positive invasive squamous cell cancer.

8.3.1 HPV–Dependent Carcinogenesis

HPV-associated SCC of the vulva develops through SIL triggered by transforming infection with high-risk HPVs, predominantly HPV 16 (Fig. 8.22). The rate of HSIL associated with HPV 16 suggests that the epithelium of the vulva may inhibit the progression of other high-risk HPV types; in contrast, in vaginal mucosa and cervical mucosa, there is greater heterogeneity of HPV types. The entry of HPV is most likely by way of skin abrasions (Fig. 8.23).

SIL mostly affects younger women. The mechanisms are similar to cervical carcinogenesis: the high-risk HPV viral gene products E6 and E7 interact with host cell p53 and Rb proteins, resulting in p53 dysfunction and inactivation of Rb, respectively. Degradation and inactivation of the tumor suppressor genes *p53* and *Rb* lead to absence of cell-cycle arrest and hyperproliferation of tumor cells. Frequent detection of overexpression for p16^{INK4a} in SIL suggests that degradation and inactivation of *p53* and *Rb* are early events in the carcinogenesis of HPV-associated SCC of the vulva. Both HPV-associated vulvar SCC and adjacent HSIL are monoclonal lesions that appear to develop from a single transformed cell.

8.3.2 HPV-Independent Carcinogenesis

Most SCCs of the vulva develop independently of HPV infection in older women through dVIN. A background of lichen sclerosus or lichen planus is common (Figs. 8.24–8.27).

The mechanism of HPV-independent carcinogenesis is not fully clear. Genetic mutations in *p53* or *PTEN* have been detected in HPV-negative vulvar SCC as well as in dVIN, suggesting that these are early changes in the HPV-independent pathway. A strong correlation between high *p53* expression and DNA aneuploidy has been reported, but not all HPV-independent vulvar SCCs follow the p53 pathway, and the pathogenesis of these tumors is unknown.

Allelic imbalance and microsatellite instability may play a role in the malignant potential of lichen sclerosus. Comparative genomic hybridization studies have shown various chromosomal alterations that might differentiate between HPV-associated and HPV-negative vulvar cancer, with HPV-positive tumors frequently showing gains of 3q and HPV-negative tumors gains of 8q. Most dVIN have a gain of 3p26. More frequent hypermethylation of *RASSF2A*, *MGMT*, and *TSP-1* genes has been found in SCC associated with lichen sclerosus than in SCC not associated with lichen sclerosus, suggesting a possible role of these genes in HPV-independent carcinogenesis.

It is unknown whether medical treatment of lichen sclerosus or lichen planus can prevent the development of dVIN and malignant transformation.

HPV-negative dVIN cannot always be attributed to lichen sclerosus or lichen planus. Also, HPV-positive SIL is sometimes seen with lichen sclerosus or lichen planus (Fig. 8.28). It is not clear whether treatment of lichen sclerosus or lichen planus with local immunosuppressive creams (corticosteroids, calcineurin inhibitors) increases the risk for HPV-associated lesions in lichen sclerosus or lichen planus.

Morbus Paget's and malignant melanoma are also independent of HPV.

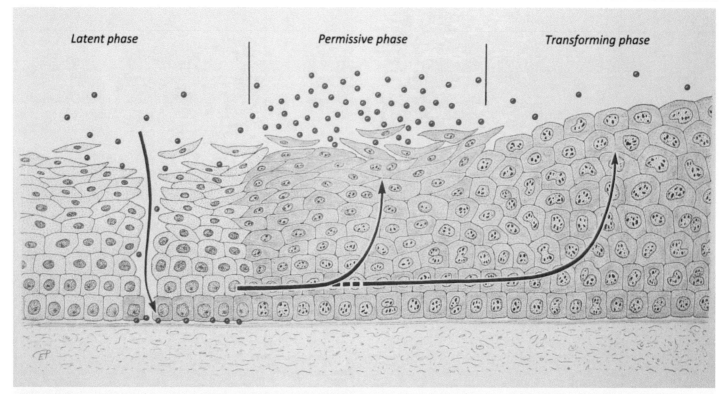

Fig. 8.23 Phases of HPV infection. Minor lacerations of the squamous epithelium permit contact of HPV with the reserve (stem) cells of the vulva. Latent infection triggers no clinical or histomorphologic changes. Permissive (productive) phase of infection can be caused by either low-risk or high-risk HPV-types. Morphologic changes correspond to condylomas or LSIL. Transforming infections of the vulva are most associated with HPV 16 and are characterized by a substantial shift of the viral gene expression profile, particularly in the basal cells. These lesions are referred to as HSIL.

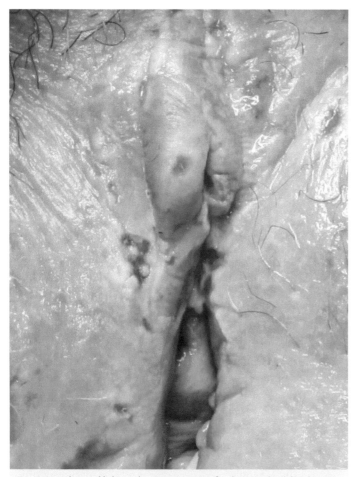

Fig. 8.24 Advanced lichen sclerosus suspicious for dVIN. Leukoplakia shows a rough and irregular surface and nonhealing erosions unresponsive to topical corticosteroids.

8.4 Preinvasive (Intraepithelial) Lesions

This group consists of SIL, dVIN, Paget's disease, and melanoma in situ.

8.4.1 Squamous Intraepithelial Lesions and Differentiated-Type Vulvar Intraepithelial Neoplasia

SIL is HPV-associated and is by far the most common preinvasive lesion of the vulvar epithelium in younger women. LSIL represents the clinical and morphologic manifestation of a productive HPV infection and is associated with low risk of malignant transformation. HSIL is a true precursor of vulvar cancer and typically corresponds to warty or basaloid-type invasive disease (Table 8.3).

SIL usually causes symptoms, mostly pain and/or pruritus. SIL can present as erythroplakia, leukoplakia, pigmented lesions, papular lesions, or erosions. These lesions are often multifocal or multicentric, with additional lesions of the cervix, vagina, or anus.

The mean time from high-risk HPV infection to development of HSIL is about 18.5 months. Spontaneous regression can occur and can be related to pregnancy. Women younger than 35 years have a higher rate of regression than older women. The risk of progression from SIL to invasive vulvar cancer is about 10% in untreated women and 3.3% in treated women. The mean interval for the progression of untreated SIL to invasion is reported to be 4 years, with almost all reported cases within 8 years.

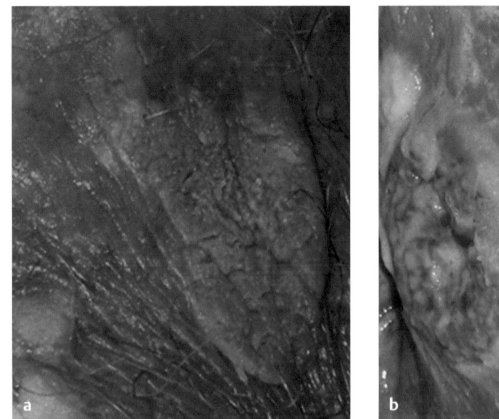

Fig. 8.25 Advanced lichen planus. (**a**) Leukoplakia with a rough and irregular surface, unresponsive to topical corticosteroids. Histology showed dVIN (**b**) followed by HPV-negative invasive cancer 6 months later.

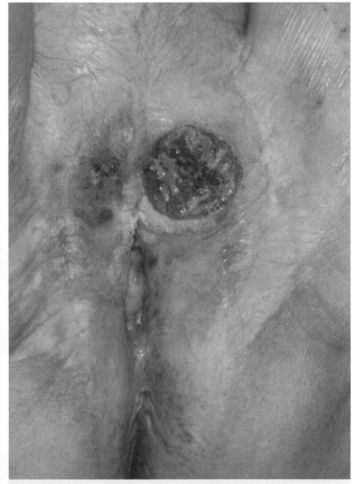

Fig. 8.26 Invasive HPV negative squamous cell cancer in a background of advanced lichen sclerosus.

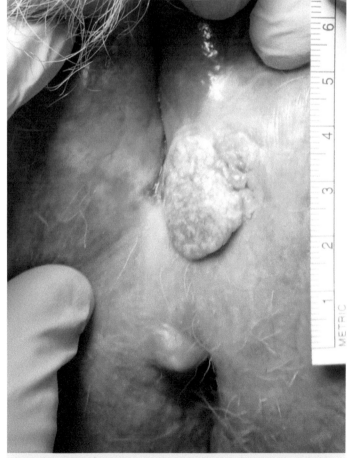

Fig. 8.27 Invasive squamous cell cancer in a background of advanced lichen planus.

Differentiated-type VIN (dVIN) is HPV-negative and typically seen in older women with long-standing and advanced lichen sclerosus or lichen planus. dVIN typically corresponds to keratinizing-type invasive disease. dVIN is by definition well differentiated and is not graded. *Differentiated* refers to the mature appearance of the epithelium, not to the grade of the lesion (Table 8.3).

The clinical diagnosis of dVIN is difficult. Symptoms are due to associated vulvar dermatoses. Leukoplakias with a rough and irregular surface, nonhealing erosions unresponsive to topical corticosteroids, or erythroplakia are suspicious and should be biopsied. Typically, lesions of dVIN do not change in appearance after application of acetic acid.

The rate of patients with lichen sclerosus or lichen planus who develop dVIN and the mean time from the manifestation of lichen sclerosus or lichen planus to dVIN are unclear. dVIN is considered more aggressive and associated with a higher and faster rate of progression to invasive carcinoma than SIL. The overall percentage of dVIN with subsequent SCC is estimated at about 33%, and the median time for progression from dVIN to SCC is about 23 months. Vulvar SCC occurring on a background of dVIN appears more likely to recur.

Management of SIL and dVIN

HSIL requires treatment, whereas LSIL can be managed expectantly. However, 30 to 42% of cases of LSIL contain high-risk HPV types and thus have the potential to progress to HSIL or invasive cancer. Treatment plans are based on colposcopy and biopsy results. Treatment of HSIL has become individualized, including different surgical modalities and medical options.

Surgical Therapy of SIL

Surgical therapy consists of ablation (Fig. 8.29) or excision (Fig. 8.30). Excision was long considered the standard of care for unifocal lesions but is more difficult for multifocal disease, which can affect large areas of the vulva. The aim is to remove all visible areas of HSIL with a 3- to 5-mm margin of normal-appearing skin. Skinning vulvectomy is considered on occasion for women with recurrent or confluent multifocal lesions. In general, more extensive surgery is associated with a greater impairment of quality of life and sexual function (Fig. 8.31).

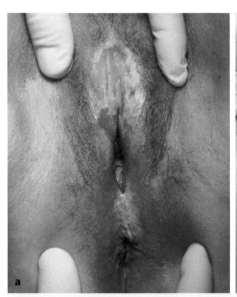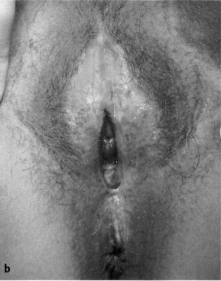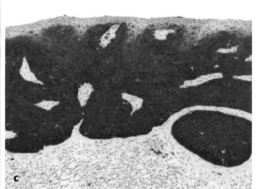

Fig. 8.28 Advanced lichen planus suspicious for HPV-positive vulvar precancer. **(a)** Note the erythroplakia and leukoplakia. **(b)** The appearance is changed after application of acetic acid. **(c)** Histology of the acetowhite epithelium shows p16^INK4a-positive HSIL, positive for HPV 16.

Table 8.3 ISSVD 2004, WHO 2003 and WHO 2014 terminologies for squamous vulva precursor lesions

ISSVD 2004	WHO 2003	WHO 2014
Condyloma	VIN 1 (mild dysplasia)	LSIL
VIN, usual type (warty, basaloid, mixed)	VIN 2 (moderate dysplasia)	HSIL
VIN, usual type (warty, basaloid, mixed)	VIN 3 (severe dysplasia, CIS)	HSIL
VIN, differentiated type	VIN, simplex type, CIS	dVIN

Abbreviations: CIS, carcinoma in situ; dVIN, differntieted-type vulvar intraepithelial neoplasia; HSIL, high-grade squamous intraepithelial lesion; ISSVD, International Society for the Study of Vulvovaginal Disease; LSIL, low-grade squamous intraepithelial lesion; VIN, vulvar intraepithelial neoplasia; WHO, World Health Organization.

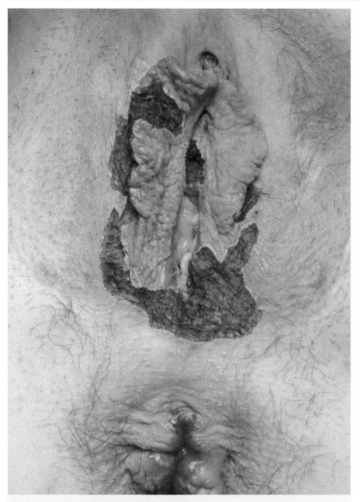

Fig. 8.29 Laser ablation of multifocal HSIL.

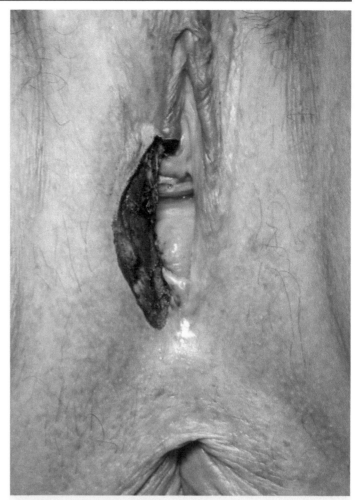

Fig. 8.30 Excision of unifocal HSIL.

Excisions are associated with positive margins in up to 66% of cases, and recurrences are common. An increased risk of recurrence has been reported in multifocal SIL compared with unifocal lesions. Recurrences have been reported in up to 19% of cases after vulvectomy, 15 to 17% after local excision with negative margins, and 46 to 50% after local excision with positive margins.

Ablation is generally performed with a CO_2 laser and can result in satisfactory results. There should be no evidence of invasion on the basis of clinical examination, colposcopy, and biopsy. As with excision, a 3- to 5-mm margin of normal-appearing skin should be treated. Occult invasive cancer (mostly with <1 mm invasion) has been reported in 3% of women undergoing surgery for SIL (Fig. 8.32). In contrast to genital condylomata, for which only superficial ablation is needed, laser ablation of HSIL requires destruction of cells through the entire thickness of the epithelium. In hair-bearing areas, laser ablation must include hair follicles, which can contain SIL and extend 3 mm or more into the subcutaneous fat. Consequently, it may be preferable to excise large lesions over hair-bearing areas. Ablation in non–hair-bearing skin should extend through the dermis (up to 2 mm). The wound can be left to heal by secondary intention, with good cosmetic results. The recurrence rate after laser vaporization is 23 to 40%.

Medical Therapy of SIL

A number of topical medical treatments have been studied for the treatment of SIL. The most widely used today are the

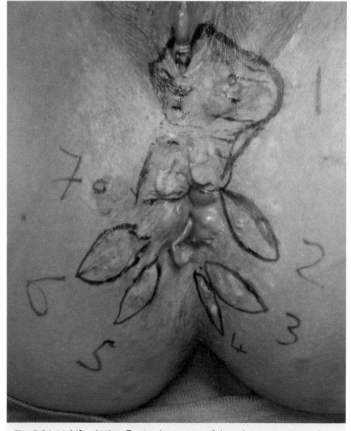

Fig. 8.31 Multifocal HSIL affecting large areas of the vulva, perineum, and perianum.

immune response modifier imiquimod and the antiviral agent cidofovir. Both can be applied in HPV-associated lesions (SIL).

Successful use of imiquimod for SIL, with response rates from 30 to 90%, has been described in a series of clinical studies including two randomized trials (Fig. 8.33). Imiquimod is applied two or three times a week, usually for 12 to 16 weeks. Regression of lesions is strongly associated with clearance of HPV. A 7-year follow-up showed a recurrence rate of 9%, which appears lower than that observed for surgical treatments. Advantages of treatment with imiquimod include enhanced clearance of HPV, self-application, and avoidance of surgery. Drawbacks of imiquimod are that it does not work in all patients, that lesions can progress during treatment potentially to invasive disease, and that local soreness, itching, and inflammation can be considerable.

Cidofovir is an antiviral agent that reduces HPV *E6* and *E7* expression and the metastatic properties of HPV-positive tumor cells. A 40% complete regression rate of SIL after topical

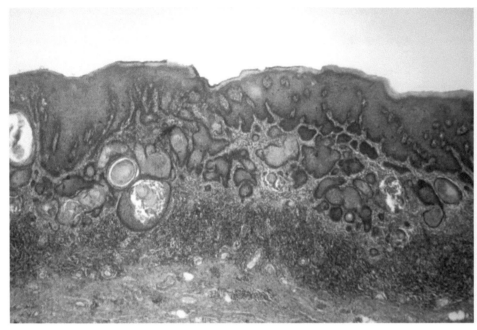

Fig. 8.32 Occult invasive cancer diagnosed histologically in an excisional specimen.

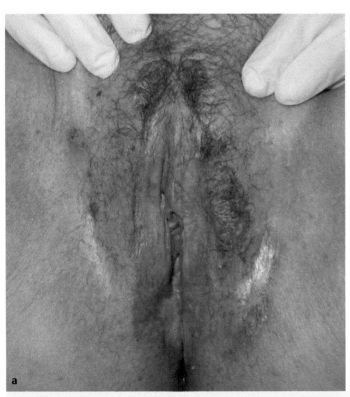

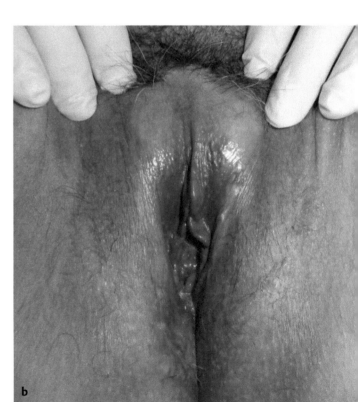

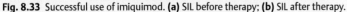

Fig. 8.33 Successful use of imiquimod. **(a)** SIL before therapy; **(b)** SIL after therapy.

application of cidofovir was reported in a series of 12 women. In our experience, cidofovir causes an intensive ulcerative reaction at the site of dVIN with no effects on the healthy skin. Cidofovir is expensive and has to be specially transferred into gel form.

Photodynamic therapy of SIL has also been used. Overall regression rate is reported to be in the range of 40 to 60%. The combination of photodynamic therapy with imiquimod is reported to have a 60% treatment response.

Therapy of dVIN

Therapy of dVIN requires surgical treatment. There is no medical treatment for dVIN and it should not be followed expectantly.

8.4.2 Paget's Disease

Paget's disease of the vulva is an uncommon intraepithelial carcinoma with erythroleukoplakic appearance. Vulvar Paget's disease arises from an intraepidermal pluripotent stem cell. Most cases occur in the epidermis and mucosa, but some invade the dermis. Paget's cells can extend into the excretory duct of sweat glands and pilosebaceous units. The risk of invasion is about 1 to 2% per year (Figs. 8.34–8.37).

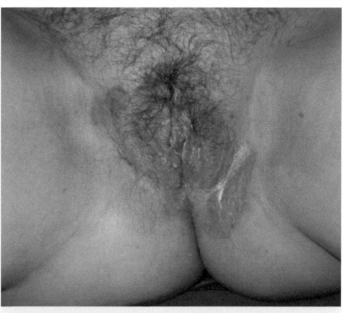

Fig. 8.34 Paget's disease with an erythroleukoplakic appearance.

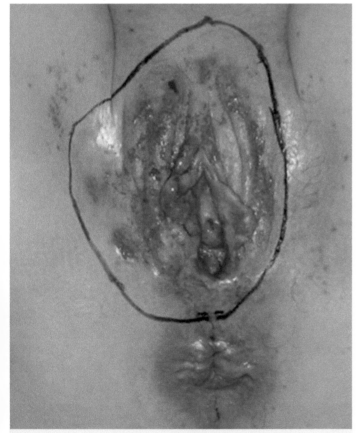

Fig. 8.35 Paget's disease with an erythroplakic appearance.

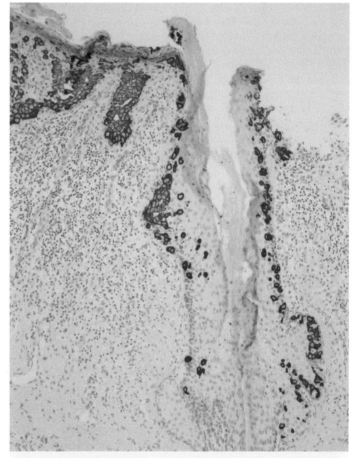

Fig. 8.36 Paget's disease. Cytokeratin-7-positive Paget's cells are distributed along the interfollicular epidermis, isthmus, infundibulum of a hair follicle, and within a sebaceous gland. (This image is provided courtesy of S. Regauer.)

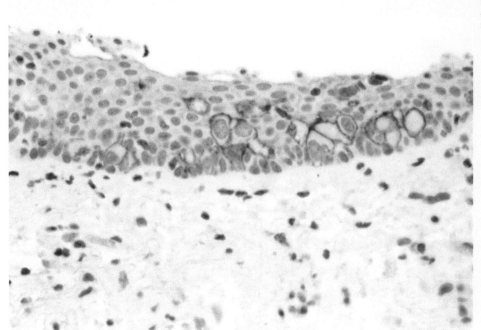

Fig. 8.37 Overexpression of p185^Her2 in Paget's disease. (This image is provided courtesy of S. Regauer.)

Diagnosis

Paget's disease can occur anywhere on the vulva, perineum, perianum, or inner thigh. The most common symptoms are itching and burning. A substantial delay between appearance of symptoms and diagnosis is common, and this is associated with larger lesions. The diagnosis is made histologically after punch biopsy. Vulvar Paget's disease can be a secondary manifestation of anal or urologic neoplasia. If the lesion extends to the urethral meatus, urethrocystoscopy should be performed; similarly, rectoscopy should be performed in patients with perianal lesions. An association of vulvar Paget's disease with synchronous malignancy at other sites now seems questionable—more due to the advanced age of these patients than to a causal association.

Treatment

Treatment of vulvar Paget's disease is challenging because of the nature of the disease and the anatomic and surgical limitations in this region. The extent of the disease is difficult to assess clinically, and surgical margins in normal-appearing skin are frequently involved histologically. Surgical excision with a 1-cm margin of normal skin is the standard treatment, but is associated with recurrence rates of up to 60%. In a retrospective series of 100 women with Paget's disease treated at eight institutions, 34% of patients developed recurrences during a follow-up of 3 years. The major problem with recurrences was extension of the disease to surrounding nongenital skin (inner thigh, perianal skin, and mons pubis), which made excision difficult. Recurrences have also been described in skin grafts from other parts of the body.

Imiquimod has reported to be effective for primary or recurrent vulvar Paget's disease in a number of small series.

8.4.3 Intraepithelial Vulvar Melanocytic Lesions and Malignant Melanoma

Pigmented vulvar lesions require biopsy because clinical examination and colposcopy cannot distinguish between benign and

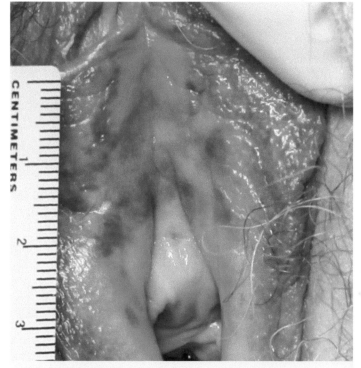

Fig. 8.38 Vulvar melanosis. The darkly pigmented macular areas have irregular borders.

malignant lesions. When sampling pigmented areas of the vulva, a biopsy should be taken of the thickest region of the lesion, or of the region with the most suspicious pattern.

Melanosis of the vulva (Fig. 8.38) is a benign lesion with increased melanin content in the keratinocytes with a slight or no increase in the number of melanocytes. These lesions are nonproliferative and are typically larger than those of genital lentigo and show brown to black pigmented macular areas with irregular borders. Normal pigmented areas can be included. Melanosis of the vulva can consist of single or multiple areas and is more common on the labia minora and the introitus.

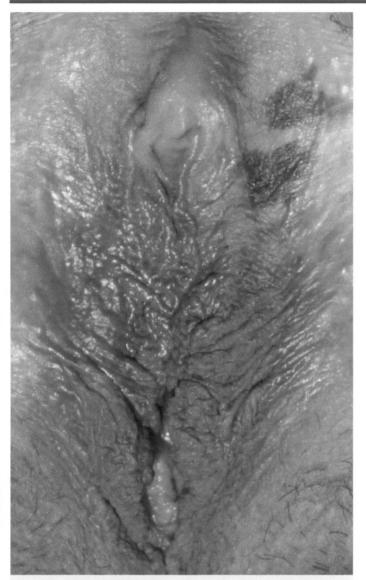

Fig. 8.39 Lentigo simplex. The figure shows two small, flat, well-demarcated, and uniformly pigmented lesions. Postinflammatory or posttraumatic pigmentation due to pigment-loaded macrophages (melanophages) can occur in obstetric scars. The specific location of this pigmentation and the presence of scars, for example, after episiotomy, are helpful in the differential diagnosis.

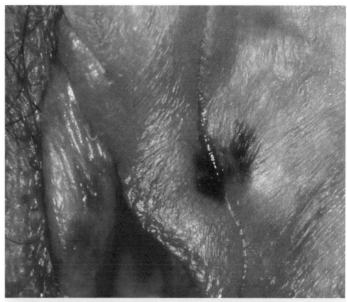

Fig. 8.40 Melanoma in situ. Darkly pigmented flat lesion in the left interlabial sulcus.

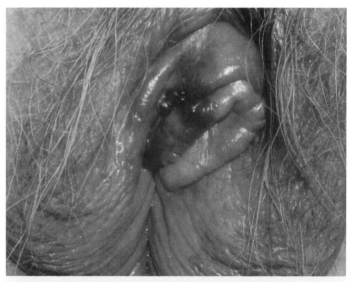

Fig. 8.41 Malignant melanoma. The dark pigmented lesion is raised.

Genital *lentigo* (Fig. 8.39) is a melanocytic cell proliferation within the basal layer. Thus, in contrast to melanosis, the number of melanocytes is increased. Clinically, these common benign lesions are typically small, flat, well demarcated, and uniformly pigmented. They can occur at all sites of the vulva. Neither melanosis nor genital lentigo forms papules or plaques. Definitive diagnosis is made by biopsy. Melanosis and genital lentigo do not require excision or ablation.

Melanocytic nevi of the vulva are uncommon. Histologically, they show a benign proliferation of nevus cells and may be junctional, compound, or intradermal. Clinically, they usually are well defined, papular, uniformly pigmented, and less than 10 mm in diameter. Atypical nevi of the vulva with prominent variable-sized junctional nests and lentiginous spread as well as dysplastic nevi with nuclear pleomorphism and irregular borders can occur, especially in young women. Nevi should be considered for excision, particularly if they change appearance or cause symptoms such as bleeding.

Malignant melanoma is the second most common malignancy of the vulva and can occur on the clitoris, labia minora, and labia majora with approximately equal frequency. Melanomas can arise de novo or from preexisting benign or atypical pigmented lesions. *Melanoma in situ* consists of malignant melanocytes that spread along the epidermis but do not extend into the papillary dermis. Clinically, these pigmented lesions are flat or slightly raised. *Invasive melanoma* not only has malignant melanocytes in the epidermis but also shows invasion in the papillary dermis. In the further course of the disease, invasion in the reticular dermis and subcutaneous fat tissue is observed. Clinically, these tumors show reddish brown to black nodules, sometimes with exulceration. Prognosis depends mostly on depth of invasion (Figs. 8.40–8.42).

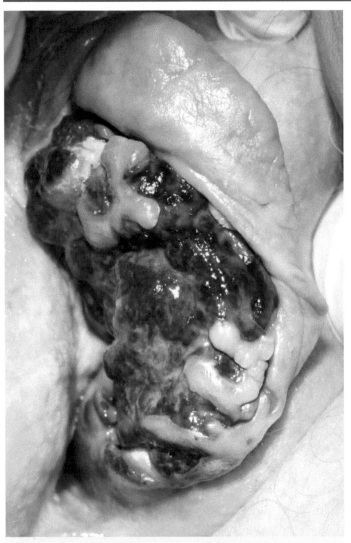

Fig. 8.42 Advanced malignant melanoma with marked nodular growth.

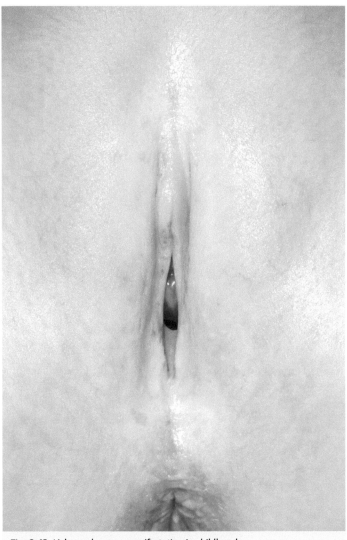

Fig. 8.43 Lichen sclerosus, manifestation in childhood.

8.5 Nonneoplastic Conditions

8.5.1 Epithelial Disorders of the Vulva

The current classification of nonneoplastic epithelial disorders of the vulva was formulated by the ISSVD in 2006. Lichen sclerosus and lichen planus are common problems and have a potential for malignant transformation. Accordingly, gynecologists should be well versed in the diagnosis, treatment, and follow-up of these conditions. Lichen sclerosus and lichen planus can have overlapping clinical and morphologic features. Further entities include lichen simplex chronicus (formerly known as *squamous hyperplasia*), psoriasis, and eczema of the vulva.

8.5.2 Lichen Sclerosus

Vulvar lichen sclerosus is a chronic localized lymphocyte-mediated dermatosis with a presumed autoimmune origin. A small percentage of patients show systemic evidence of T-cell immune deficiencies. If the condition is untreated over many years, progressive sclerosis results in scarring with severe distortion of the normal vulvar anatomy. The condition can occur in childhood (Figs. 8.43 and 8.44).

The cardinal symptoms of lichen sclerosus are intractable vulvar itching and soreness. Lichen sclerosus begins with uncharacteristic pruritus, burning, dysuria, dyspareunia, and pain. Early symptoms are often ignored or interpreted as secondary effects of yeast infections. Thus, patients with persistent vulvar symptoms should be evaluated by biopsy

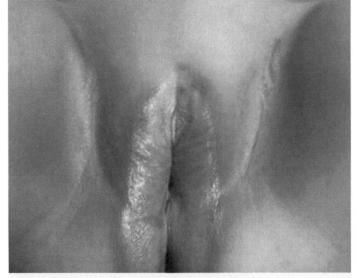

Fig. 8.44 Lichen sclerosus, manifestation in childhood.

early. Early lichen sclerosus (Figs. 8.45–8.47) often affects the periclitoral area and then spreads to the interlabial sulci. Early lichen sclerosus can show prominent shiny erythema, mild depigmentation, thinning of the mucosa, and mild asymmetry of the labia minora. Quite often, lichen sclerosus involves the perineum and the perianal skin in a figure-of-8 distribution. Many patients have slow progression over years (Figs. 8.48 and

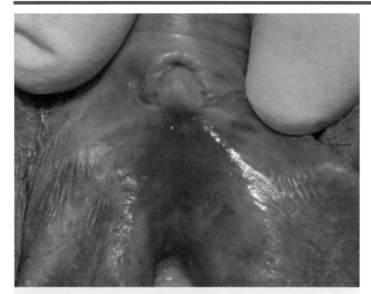

Fig. 8.45 Early lichen sclerosus affecting the periclitoral area. Note the prominent shiny erythema and thinning of the mucosa.

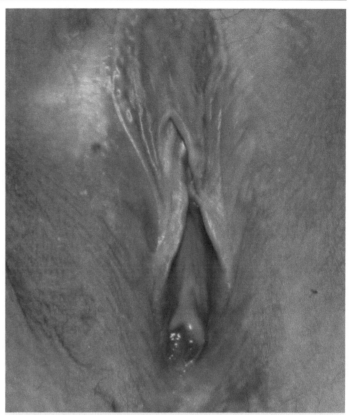

Fig. 8.46 Early lichen sclerosus with spread to the interlabial sulci. Note the mild depigmentation and mild asymmetry of the labia minora.

8.49) with multiple complete or partial remissions. Late lichen sclerosus (Figs. 8.50 and 8.51) associated with destructive scarring, depigmentation, progressive loss of the labia minora, synechiae, and vaginal stenosis (kraurosis vulvae in the old literature) carries significant morbidity. Progression can be prevented with consistent treatment and follow-up. SCCs develop in 3 to 5% of patients with long-standing and untreated vulvar lichen sclerosus. It is unknown whether early diagnosis and treatment of lichen sclerosus and lichen planus reduce the risk of malignant transformation.

First-line treatment of lichen sclerosus with a superpotent topical corticosteroid has a high response rate. A suitable regimen is clobetasol propionate 0.05% ointment once daily for 1 month, alternate days for 1 month, and twice weekly for 1 month, then reducing to as needed. A 30-g tube should last about 3 months, and for most patients it will last longer. A similar regimen may be used in children. Potential side effects of corticoid therapy include cutaneous atrophy or adrenal suppression, but in practice and with careful monitoring, these side effects are rare. Local indifferent ointments should be used to minimize local steroid side effects.

Second-line therapies include topical calcineurin inhibitors: pimecrolimus and tacrolimus have been demonstrated to be effective. This type of treatment works exclusively through interactions with lymphocytes in active stages of disease.

8.5.3 Lichen Planus

Lichen planus is a mucocutaneous disease of unknown origin that can involve the skin, oral mucosa, genitalia, esophagus, and skin appendages. There are three main clinical types: classic, erosive, and hypertrophic (Figs. 8.52–8.54). As in lichen sclerosus, the etiology of lichen planus is probably immunologic, with T cells activated by an as yet unknown antigen to attack the basal keratinocytes. There appears to be an association with hepatitis C, and patients with lichen planus should be tested accordingly.

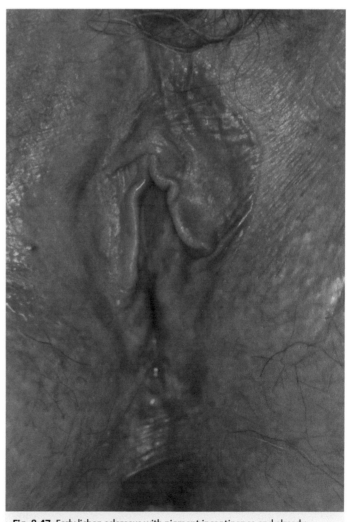

Fig. 8.47 Early lichen sclerosus with pigment incontinence and already considerably reduced labia minora.

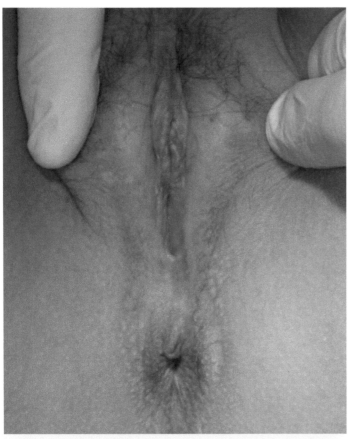

Fig. 8.48 Intermediate lichen sclerosus involving the perineum and perianal skin.

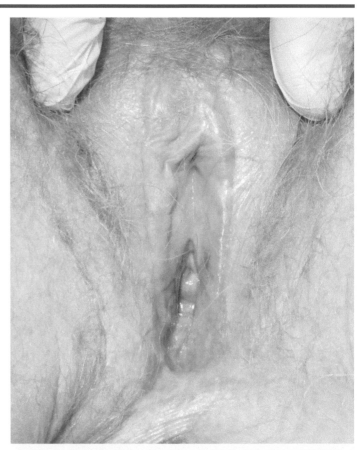

Fig. 8.49 Intermediate lichen sclerosus. Note the depigmentation of the labia minora and interlabial sulci.

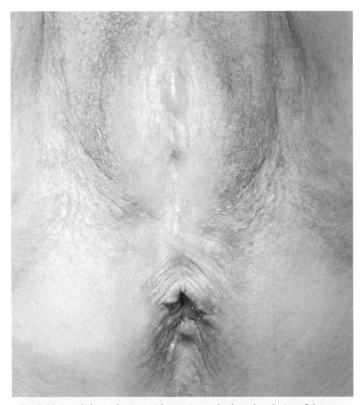

Fig. 8.50 Late lichen sclerosus with scarring and subtotal occlusion of the introitus.

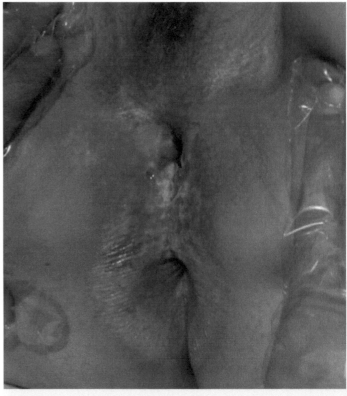

Fig. 8.51 End-stage lichen sclerosus. The anatomy of the vulva is severely distorted.

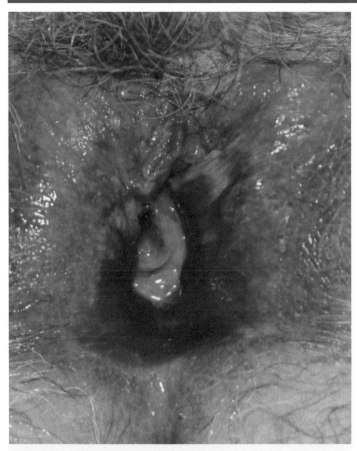

Fig. 8.52 Lichen planus with vaginal involvement.

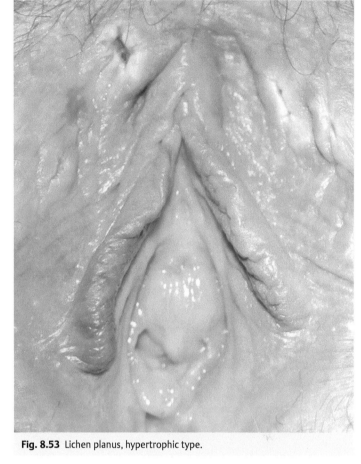

Fig. 8.53 Lichen planus, hypertrophic type.

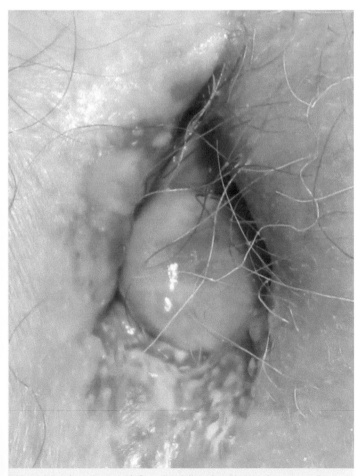

Fig. 8.54 Lichen planus with fine whitish lines (Wickham's phenomenon).

Patients with genital lichen planus usually have severe pruritus and soreness. Lichen planus affecting the mucosal side of the vulva typically involves the inner aspects of the labia minora and consists of a glazed erythema that may easily bleed on touching and fine whitish lines, the Wickham's phenomenon. Erosions may develop. In later stage, lichen planus commonly leads to a reduction and fusion of the labia minora and vagina. This may result in a buried clitoris and urethra, a narrow vaginal introitus, and a fused vagina, making penetration impossible.

In contrast to lichen sclerosus, genital lichen planus typically involves the vaginal mucosa. Patients with genital lichen planus should be examined for other mucosal lesions, in particular in the mouth. The vulvovaginal-gingival syndrome is a subgroup of lichen planus and can be a multisystem disorder.

The exact incidence of malignancy associated with lichen planus is unknown. It is unknown whether early diagnosis and treatment of lichen sclerosus and lichen planus reduce the risk of malignant transformation.

The treatment of lichen planus is similar to that of lichen sclerosus. Clobetasol propionate (0.05%) ointment is effective. Foam preparations can be used for vaginal lesions. Calcineurin inhibitors pimecrolimus and tacrolimus are second-line options.

8.5.4 Psoriasis

Psoriasis is a chronic inflammatory skin disease with accelerated epidermal proliferation and disturbed differentiation. There is no increased risk of secondary malignancy. Psoriasis is most commonly seen on the elbows, knees, scalp, and nails but can also occur on the vulva. Clinical features include silvery scaling and sharply demarcated erythema. The erythema and sharp outline tend to remain, and fissuring is seen. In contrast to lichen sclerosus and lichen planus, psoriasis often involves the labia majora

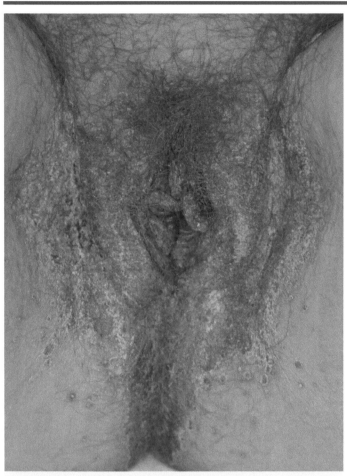

Fig. 8.55 Psoriasis with silvery scaling and sharply demarcated erythema. Note the involvement of the labia majora which usually does not occur in lichen sclerosus and lichen planus.

(Fig. 8.55). This can be helpful in the differential diagnosis. Vulvar psoriasis initially is treated with a potent steroid and a vitamin D ointment, always in consultation with a dermatologist.

8.5.5 Lichen Simplex

Lichen simplex describes a dermatologic affection seen on the apparently normal vulva secondary to chronic itching and rubbing. The term *lichen simplex chronicus* is used when the lichenification develops as a palpable thickening with increased prominence of skin markings on skin that had been previously normal in appearance and where other disorders (i.e., lichen sclerosus, lichen planus, psoriasis) have been ruled out. The term *lichenification* is used for similar changes on a background of a visible dermatosis. Lichen simplex chronicus is characterized by an intractable itch–scratch cycle. Lichen simplex chronicus is more common in women with allergies and atopic dermatitis at other sites. Itching normally responds quickly to application of a potent topical steroid to break the itch–scratch

cycle. A sedating antihistamine such as hydroxyzine may be helpful at night.

8.5.6 Vulvar Eczema

Vulvar eczemas can be classified as atopic eczema, irritant contact dermatitis (from topical treatments, cosmetic preparations, wet wipes, and mechanical friction from sanitary pads), and allergic contact dermatitis (from delayed-type or cell-mediated immunity). Especially atopic vulvar eczema is characterized by severe itching and lichenification. Known allergens are anesthetics, antibiotics, anticandidal agents, antiseptics, corticosteroids, and spermicides as medications. Additional agents, among others, are cosmetics, preservatives, fragrances, emollients, panty liners, snaps, buckles, pins, and clothing. Patch testing should be done to identify relevant allergens, and causative agents should be withdrawn and irritative stimuli avoided. In case of atopic eczema, patients should be referred to dermatologists. Topical steroids are prescribed according to severity.

Further Reading

Bergeron C, Ferenczy A, Richart RM, Guralnick M. Micropapillomatosis labialis appears unrelated to human papillomavirus. Obstet Gynecol 1990;76:281–286

Bornstein J, Sideri M, Tatti S, Walker P, Prendiville W, Haefner HK; Nomenclature Committee of International Federation for Cervical Pathology and Colposcopy. 2011 terminology of the vulva of the International Federation for Cervical Pathology and Colposcopy. J Low Genit Tract Dis 2012;16:290–295

Bornstein J, Bogliatto F, Haefner HK, et al; ISSVD Terminology Committee. The 2015 International Society for the Study of Vulvovaginal Disease (ISSVD) Terminology of Vulvar Squamous Intraepithelial Lesions. Obstet Gynecol 2016;127:264–268

Cheng S, Kirtschig G, Cooper S, Thornhill M, Leonardi-Bee J, Murphy R. Interventions for erosive lichen planus affecting mucosal sites. Cochrane Database Syst Rev 2012;2:CD008092

Chi CC, Kirtschig G, Baldo M, Brackenbury F, Lewis F, Wojnarowska F. Topical interventions for genital lichen sclerosus. Cochrane Database Syst Rev 2011;12:CD008240

Jones RW, Rowan DM, Stewart AW. Vulvar intraepithelial neoplasia: aspects of the natural history and outcome in 405 women. Obstet Gynecol 2005;106:1319–1326

Le Cleach L, Chosidow O. Clinical practice. Lichen planus. N Engl J Med 2012;366: 723–732

Mathiesen O, Buus SK, Cramers M. Topical imiquimod can reverse vulvar intraepithelial neoplasia: a randomised, double-blinded study. Gynecol Oncol 2007;107:219–222

Pepas L, Kaushik S, Bryant A, Nordin A, Dickinson HO. Medical interventions for high grade vulval intraepithelial neoplasia. Cochrane Database Syst Rev 2011;13:CD007924

Polterauer S, Catharina Dressler A, Grimm C, et al. Accuracy of preoperative vulva biopsy and the outcome of surgery in vulvar intraepithelial neoplasia 2 and 3. Int J Gynecol Pathol 2009;28:559–562

Regauer S, Eberz B, Reich O. Human-Papillomavirus induced squamous intraepithelial lesions in vulvar lichen planus. J Low Gen Tract Dis 2016 (in press)

Regauer S, Reich O, Eberz B. Vulvar cancers in women with vulvar lichen planus: a clinico-pathological study. J Am Acad Dermatol 2014;71:698–707

Regauer S. Extramammary Paget's disease—a proliferation of adnexal origin? Histopathology 2006;48:723–729

Regauer S. Residual anogenital lichen sclerosus after cancer surgery has a high risk for recurrence: a clinicopathological study of 75 women. Gynecol Oncol 2011;123:289–294

Terlou A, van Seters M, Ewing PC, et al. Treatment of vulvar intraepithelial neoplasia with topical imiquimod: seven years median follow-up of a randomized clinical trial. Gynecol Oncol 2011;121:157–162

van Seters M, van Beurden M, de Craen AJ. Is the assumed natural history of vulvar intraepithelial neoplasia III based on enough evidence? A systematic review of 3322 published patients. Gynecol Oncol 2005;97:645–651

Kurman RJ, Carcangiu ML, Herrington CS, Young RH, eds. World Health Organization Classification of Tumours of the Female Reproductive Organs. 4th ed. Lyon: IARC Press; 2014

Chapter 9

Colposcopy of the Vagina

9 Colposcopy of the Vagina

9.1 Histology

The squamous mucosa lining the vagina is similar to the original squamous epithelium of the cervix. Embryologically, the epithelium of the distal vagina appears to be derived from the epithelium of the urogenital sinus epithelium, which is itself of endodermal origin, whereas the epithelium of the upper vagina is of mesodermal müllerian origin. The vaginal stroma is composed of a mixture of elastic fibers and can contain mesonephric or wolffian remnants. The persistence of glands arising from müllerian epithelium (so-called vaginal adenosis) is uncommon, and the vagina usually does not contain glands.

9.2 Vaginal Carcinogenesis

The large majority of malignant vaginal neoplasms are squamous cell carcinomas that develop via squamous intraepithelial lesions (SILs; formerly vaginal intraepithelial neoplasia, or VAIN) associated with human papillomavirus (HPV) infection. Patients with risk factors for persisting HPV infection (e.g., smoking, immunosuppression, HIV infection) have an increased risk for vaginal precancer and cancer. Occasional squamous cell carcinomas of the vagina may develop in a background of lichen planus independently of HPV infection. The mechanism of HPV-independent carcinogenesis of the vagina seems to parallel that of the vulva.

9.3 Squamous Intraepithelial Lesions

SIL of the vagina accounts for less than 1% of lower genital tract intraepithelial neoplasia. Women with vaginal SIL are usually asymptomatic. The first report of SIL is credited to Graham and Meigs in patients years after treatment for carcinoma in situ of the cervix. Vaginal SIL can occur alone or as synchronously or metachronously with cervical or vulvar HPV-related precancer and cancer. Up to 65% of patients with vaginal SIL have been reported to have SIL of the cervix or vulva.

Lesions are often multifocal and occur predominantly in the upper one-third of the vagina, whereas the middle and lower thirds are involved in less than 10%. This is probably due to the dual origin of vaginal epithelium during prenatal development.

Most lower-grade SILs probably regress spontaneously. In contrast, untreated higher-grade SILs progress to invasive cancer in 5 to 8% of cases.

9.4 Diagnostic Methods for SIL

9.4.1 History

A history of SIL of the cervix is a major risk factor for the development of vaginal SIL. About 0.9 to 7.4% of patients with hysterectomy for cervical SIL later develop vaginal SIL. Vaginal SIL can develop as an independent lesion or close to the cervix (or vaginal apex after hysterectomy). Patients with residual SIL at the vaginal apex after hysterectomy appear at risk of developing invasive vaginal cancer.

As for other HPV-related neoplasias, smoking is a risk factor for vaginal carcinoma. Vaginal SIL is also known to occur more frequently in patients with a history of pelvic radiation for other malignancies such as cervical or endometrial cancer. This increased incidence of vaginal SIL may take some 10 to 15 years to manifest itself. Possible mechanisms of postradiation cellular dysplasia include radiation-induced expression of HPV oncoproteins and radiation-induced changes in the cellular response to HPV infection.

Vaginal adenosis is any condition in which columnar epithelium exists within the vagina. Metaplasia can convert this glandular epithelium to squamous epithelium. It is unclear whether high-risk HPV-infected women with vaginal adenosis are at greater risk for vaginal high-grade squamous intraepithelial lesion (HSIL). Vaginal adenosis may be the origin of the rare entities of vaginal adenoma and adenocarcinoma.

9.4.2 Colposcopy of the Vagina

In many cases, vaginal SIL cannot be identified by gross inspection only; colposcopy of the vagina is essential. Particularly, women who have positive cytology after treatment for cervical SIL should be examined carefully for vaginal SIL. At the examination, it is important to rotate the open duckbill speculum through 360 degrees, paying particular attention to the upper vagina. In the posthysterectomy patient, vaginal vault angles can be dimpled, precluding complete colposcopic assessment.

After application of acetic acid, vaginal SIL is usually acetowhite with sharp borders and a granular surface appearance (Fig. 9.1). Occasionally, there is a punctation. Mosaic or keratosis is rarely found. The colposcopic appearance of vaginal SIL can be different from that of cervical intraepithelial neoplasia (CIN) and may manifest only as iodine-yellow epithelium. Thus, the application of iodine is important. After iodine, vaginal SIL usually stains light yellow (Fig. 9.2). Interpretation of Lugol's test can be difficult in postmenopausal patients with atrophy. The application of a topical estrogen for up to 3 to 4 weeks can be helpful.

The 2011 International Federation of Cervical Pathology and Colposcopy (IFCPC) colposcopic terminology of the vagina distinguishes minor and major lesions, so as to improve the correlation with histology and implications for treatment. Atypical and fragile vessels and lesions with an irregular surface and ulceration are suspicious for invasive disease (Fig. 9.3)

The vagina is frequently involved by advanced primary cancers of neighboring organs such as the cervix, vulva, and rectum (Figs. 9.4 and 9.5).

9.4.3 Cytology

Persisting abnormal cervical cytology in a patient with a colposcopically normal cervix should prompt exact inspection of the vagina. Although patients with the cytologic changes of low-grade squamous intraepithelial lesion (LSIL) may not have an identifiable lesion, cytologic findings of HSIL generally are associated with a corresponding colposcopic and histologic lesion.

9.4.4 Biopsy

Biopsy should be performed on any visible lesions to define the diagnosis and rule out invasion. Injection of local anesthetic is usually not necessary. Histologic examination can also be performed with abrasion of vaginal mucosal fragments. We use small sieves to avoid losing small mucosal fragments (Fig. 9.6).

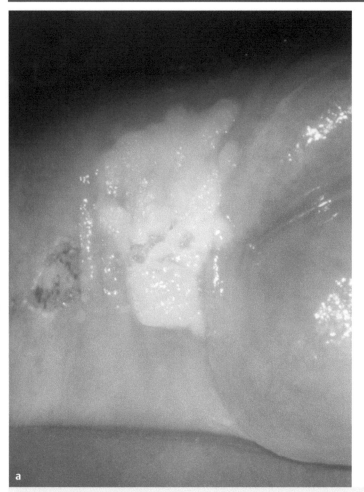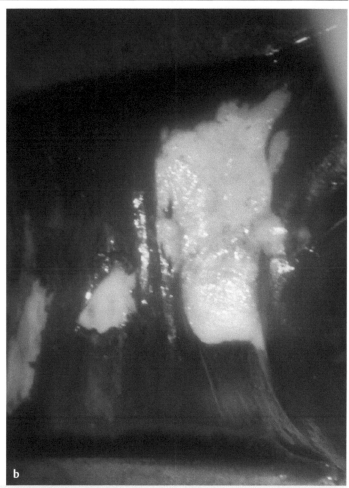

Fig. 9.1 Vaginal HSIL **(a)** before and **(b)** after Lugol's solution. The small erosion next to the lesion is an artifact caused by the speculum.

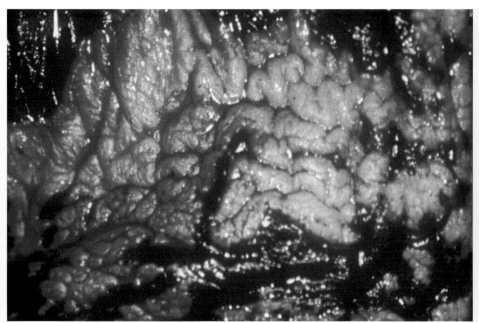

Fig. 9.2 Vaginal HSIL after Lugol's solution. The slightly elevated lesions stain light yellow.

9.4.5 Biomarkers

Differentiating between low-risk and high-risk HPV infection is important because LSIL containing HPV 6 or 11 is histologically indistinguishable from LSIL associated with high-risk HPVs. It may well be that only high-risk HPV infections have the potential to induce HSIL and invasive disease. HPV testing is also used in the follow-up of patients treated for vaginal SIL.

Staining for p16^{INK4a} with or without Ki-67 can be helpful to triage HPV-induced SIL and avoid overtreatment. SIL with negative staining tends to regress, whereas SIL with positive staining denotes transforming HPV infection. These lesions trend to persist or progress (Fig. 9.7).

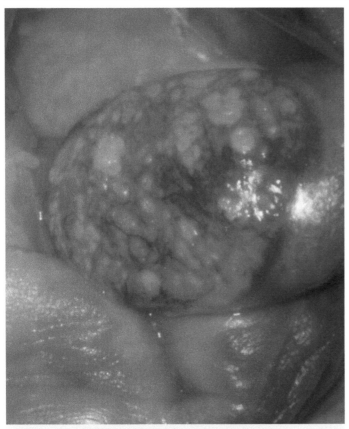

Fig. 9.3 Invasive vaginal cancer. Note the evident atypical vessels.

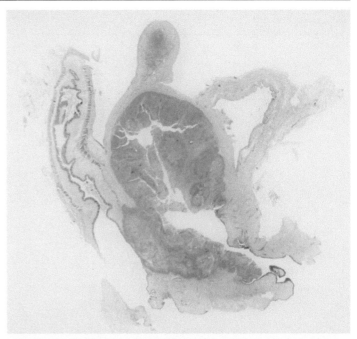

Fig. 9.4 Cervical cancer with extensive infiltration of the vagina. Giant frontal section of an exenteration specimen.

9.5 Histologic Terminology and Classification

The WHO has adapted the 2014 classification of vaginal lesions accordingly as LSIL (formerly mild dysplasia) and HSIL (formerly VAIN 2/3, carcinoma in situ).

9.6 Histomorphology of Vaginal SIL

The microscopic features of vaginal SIL are analogous to those of CIN (SIL). The spectrum of vaginal SIL includes lesions classified as condylomas (LSIL of the vagina, VAIN 1) and lesions classified as high-grade vaginal intraepithelial neoplasia (HSIL of the vagina, VAIN 2 and 3). Histologically, LSIL of the vagina parallels CIN I and includes exophytic and flat condyloma. HSIL of the vagina is characterized by nuclear abnormalities including enlargement with irregular shape, hyperchromasia, and irregular condensation of chromatin at all levels of the epithelium. Increased mitotic activity with abnormal figures, acanthosis, and dyskeratosis occurs. The differential diagnosis includes atrophy, radiation changes, and immature squamous metaplasia in women with vaginal adenosis.

9.7 Management of SIL

Treatment is planned according to the number, extent, and location of lesions, their grade, and previous treatments as well as patient age and preference. HPV testing with p16^{INK4a} staining is helpful.

9.7.1 LSIL of the Vagina

LSIL often regresses and most often is not associated with neoplastic transformation. Expectant management can be appropriate initially. Patients with nonsuspicious colposcopy of the vagina and only mild cytologic abnormalities do not require treatment.

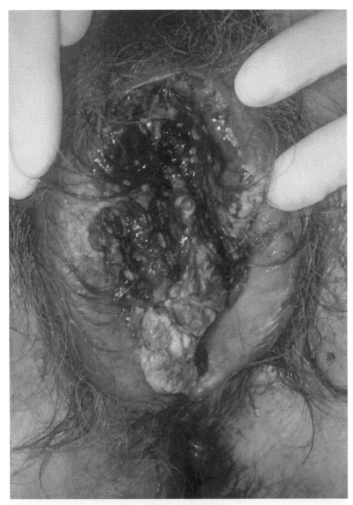

Fig. 9.5 Vulval cancer with infiltration of the vagina.

normal-appearing mucosa. The major advantage of laser ablation is the ability to control the depth and width of ablation under direct vision through the colposcope. As the thickness of the vaginal epithelium affected by SIL is 0.1 to 1.4 mm, vaporization should be done to a depth of 2 mm. In patients after hysterectomy with lesions located in the dimples of the vaginal vault, excision should be considered prior to ablation to rule out occult invasive cancer. If a larger area is involved, a partial colpectomy (vaginectomy) can be indicated.

Invasion should be ruled out as far as possible before ablative therapy

Surgery is successful in about 70 to 80% of cases. HSIL following radiation may be more refractory to treatment, more likely to recur, and more likely to progress to invasive cancer than HSIL not associated with radiation therapy.

9.7.4 Medical Therapy

Imiquimod is effective in the management of vaginal SIL in the background of HPV infection and is helpful for multifocal lesions. Our practice is to use imiquimod 2.5% vaginal suppositories (week 1 and 2: one vaginal suppository per week; week 3 and 4: two vaginal suppositories per week; after week 5: three suppositories per week for a maximum of 16 weeks). Patients need to be counseled regarding side effects (flulike symptoms, fever) and off-label use.

Treatment with 5-fluorouracil (5-FU) cream has been reported as an option for VAIN after radiation, VAIN in immunocompromised women, and multifocal VAIN refractory to imiquimod and too extensive to treat with laser vaporization. Usually 1 to 2 mL of 5% 5-FU cream is administered once a week under close observation and stopped when the surface of the lesion peels away. The major complication with 5-FU is sloughing of the vaginal epithelium that will not heal.

9.7.5 Other Treatment Modalities

Electrocoagulation of SIL can lead to vaginal stenosis and is not recommended.

Loop excision is considered contraindicated because of the risk of perforation of the vagina. Radiotherapy has a limited role in the primary treatment but has a role in refractory cases and as an adjunct to surgery in early invasive carcinoma. Interferon injection and cavitational ultrasonic surgical aspiration have also been proposed for the treatment of vaginal SIL.

Patients after treatment for preinvasive disease retain a risk for developing invasive disease (in the 2–5% range) and should be followed up accordingly. We follow up with patients after treatment of vaginal HSIL with Pap tests and colposcopy every 6 months for at least 2 years. HPV testing is an additional method to predict the persistence or recurrence of disease after treatment.

9.8 Vaginal Melanoma

Vaginal melanoma (invasive and in situ) is rare. As a mucosal melanoma, its biology and behavior are distinct from that of cutaneous melanoma. Amelanotic lesions may be detected on the basis of abnormal cytology and colposcopy (Fig. 9.8). Invasive vaginal melanoma is frequently multifocal and has a substantial in situ component, which renders complete surgical resection difficult. Local and distant recurrences are common even when negative margins are achieved. Outcomes are poor.

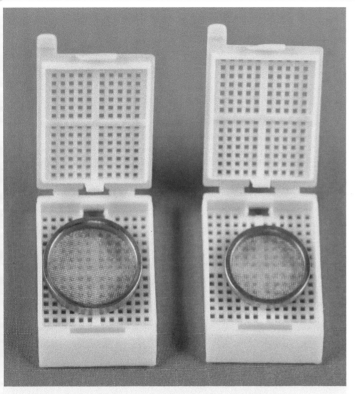

Fig. 9.6 Small sieves for histologic processing of vaginal abrasions.

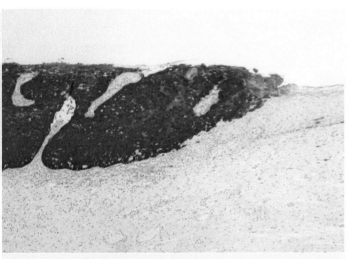

Fig. 9.7 p16^{INK4a}-positive HSIL of the vagina.

Patients can follow up with a Pap test and colposcopy every 6 months. If associated with high-risk HPV, LSIL can progress.

9.7.2 HSIL of the Vagina

HSIL requires treatment. Up to 10 to 28% of patients are subsequently found to have early invasion.

9.7.3 Surgical Therapy

Surgical modalities include excision and ablation. The aim is to remove all visibly affected areas with a 3- to 5-mm margin of

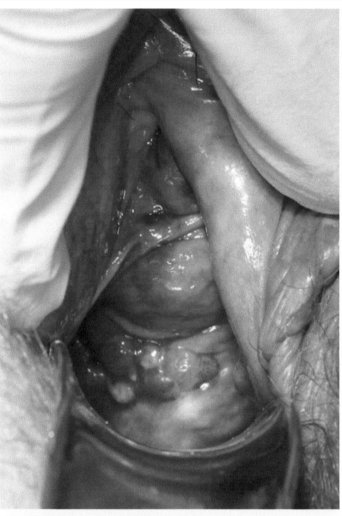

Fig. 9.8 Amelanotic melanoma of the vagina.

Further Reading

Benedet JL, Wilson PS, Matisic JP. Epidermal thickness measurements in vaginal intraepithelial neoplasia. A basis for optimal CO2 laser vaporization. J Reprod Med 1992;37:809–812

Bornstein J, Bentley J, Bösze P, et al. 2011 colposcopic terminology of the International Federation for Cervical Pathology and Colposcopy. Obstet Gynecol 2012;120(1):166–172

Chiu TL, Jones RW. Multifocal multicentric squamous cell carcinomas arising in vulvovaginal lichen planus. J Low Genit Tract Dis 2011;15:246–247

Diakomanolis E, Haidopoulos D, Stefanidis K. Treatment of high-grade vaginal intraepithelial neoplasia with imiquimod cream. N Engl J Med 2002;347:374

Dodge JA, Eltabbakh GH, Mount SL, Walker RP, Morgan A. Clinical features and risk of recurrence among patients with vaginal intraepithelial neoplasia. Gynecol Oncol 2001;83:363–369

Frumovitz M, Etchepareborda M, Sun CC, et al. Primary malignant melanoma of the vagina. Obstet Gynecol 2010;116:1358–1365

Gurumurthy M, Cruickshank ME. Management of vaginal intraepithelial neoplasia. J Low Genit Tract Dis 2012;16:306–312

Indermaur MD, Martino MA, Fiorica JV, Roberts WS, Hoffman MS. Upper vaginectomy for the treatment of vaginal intraepithelial neoplasia. Am J Obstet Gynecol 2005;193:577–580, discussion 580–581

Kurman RJ, Carcangiu ML, Herrington CS, Young RH, eds. WHO Classification of Tumors of the Female Reproductive Organs. 4th ed. Lyon: IARC Press; 2014

Liao JB, Jean S, Wilkinson-Ryan I, et al. Vaginal intraepithelial neoplasia (VAIN) after radiation therapy for gynecologic malignancies: a clinically recalcitrant entity. Gynecol Oncol 2011;120:108–112

Reich O, Fritsch H. The developmental origin of cervical and vaginal epithelium and their clinical consequences: a systematic review. J Low Genit Tract Dis 2014;18:358–360

Rome RM, England PG. Management of vaginal intraepithelial neoplasia: a series of 132 cases with long-term follow-up. Int J Gynecol Cancer 2000;10:382–390

Schockaert S, Poppe W, Arbyn M, Verguts T, Verguts J. Incidence of vaginal intraepithelial neoplasia after hysterectomy for cervical intraepithelial neoplasia: a retrospective study. Am J Obstet Gynecol 2008;199:113.e1–113.e5

Song JH, Lee JH, Lee JH, et al. High-dose-rate brachytherapy for the treatment of vaginal intraepithelial neoplasia. Cancer Res Treat 2014;46:74–80

Wentz WB, Reagan JW. Clinical significance of postirradiation dysplasia of the uterine cervix. Am J Obstet Gynecol 1970;106:812–817

Zeligs KP, Byrd K, Tarney CM, et al. A clinicopathologic study of vaginal intraepithelial neoplasia. Obstet Gynecol 2013;122:1223–1230

Chapter 10

Colposcopy of the Perianal Region

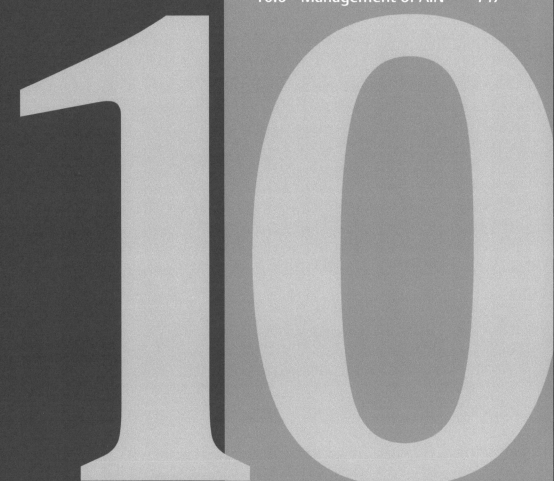

10 Colposcopy of the Perianal Region

10.1 Anatomy and Histology

The anus consists of the anal canal and the anal margin. The anal canal begins at the apex of the anal sphincter complex, where the rectum enters the puborectalis sling, and ends with the squamous mucosa blending with the perianal skin. This roughly coincides with the palpable intersphincteric groove. Immediately proximal to the dentate line, a narrow zone of transitional mucosa is variably present—the anal transformation zone (TZ). Distal to this, the mucosa consists of squamous epithelium devoid of hairs and glands. The anal margin extends distal to the anal verge (the junction of the hair-bearing skin) (Fig. 10.1).

10.2 Anal Carcinogenesis

About 80% of anal cancers are of squamous cell origin, with the remainder being adenocarcinomas. More than 85% of anal cancers are associated with human papillomavirus (HPV) and develop via anal intraepithelial neoplasia (AIN). In HPV-associated anal cancer, HPV 16 predominates, followed by HPV 18, as well as HPV 33 and HPV 59.

The entry of HPV is most likely by way of skin abrasions. Anal intercourse is a likely risk factor. The proximity of the vaginal introitus to the anus also facilitates nonsexual and autoinoculation in women via vaginal secretions, digital transfer, or transfer of fomites. Women with other HPV-related gynecologic neoplasms are at increased risk for developing anal cancer.

A minority of squamous cell carcinomas of the anus develop independently of HPV in a background of lichen sclerosus or lichen planus (Fig. 10.2). The mechanism of HPV-independent carcinogenesis of the anus has not yet been elucidated but seems to parallel that of the vulva (Fig. 10.3).

Topographically, anal cancers are located in the anal canal or, to a lesser extent, at the anal margin. Most anal cancers originate from the anal TZ (linea dentata) of the anal canal.

10.3 Anal Intraepithelial Neoplasia

The AIN lesions can be intra-anal or perianal. AIN can involve the anal canal by extending from the perianal skin inward or into the canal in isolation. Thus, evidence of perianal HPV infection must prompt the possibility of AIN within the anal canal. More than 75% of AIN lesions are located on the anal TZ. Risk factors are unprotected receptive anal intercourse, lifetime number of sexual partners, a history of genital warts, immunodeficiency, smoking, and a history of HPV-related gynecologic neoplasm including vulvar intraepithelial neoplasia (VIN) and cervical intraepithelial neoplasia (CIN).

AIN can also present as part of a multifocal disease process involving any or all anogenital sites (Fig. 10.4). In a study of immunocompetent women with CIN, VIN, or vaginal intraepithelial neoplasia, 12% had AIN and 8% had high-grade (HG)-AIN. Another study of immunocompetent women found AIN in 17% of women with CIN, with 4% having HG-AIN. Interestingly, patients with multiple lesions in different areas of the female genital tract often show the same HPV type in all of the lesions.

HPV 16, 18, 33, and 58 are the types most frequently detected in HG-AIN. The prevalence of multiple-type infections decreased from 54% in low-grade (LG)-AIN 1 to 7% in anal carcinoma.

The rate of progression from LG-AIN to HG-AIN is reported to be 36 to 66% over 2 years; the rate of progression from HG-AIN to invasive anal cancer has been reported as 5 to 26% over 5 years.

Patients with AIN report pruritus and burning sensations or are asymptomatic. Clinically, AIN can present as erythroplakia,

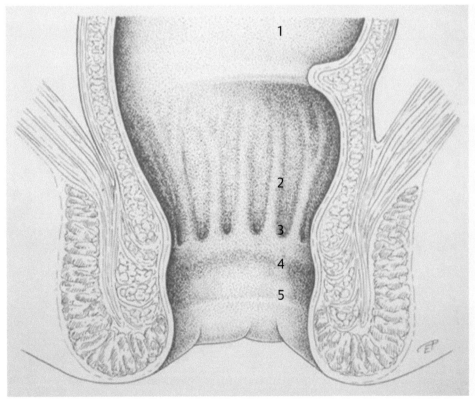

Fig. 10.1 Anatomy of the anus. **1** Rectum; **2** anal transformation zone with columns of Morgagni; **3** dentate line; **4** anal canal; **5** anal margin.

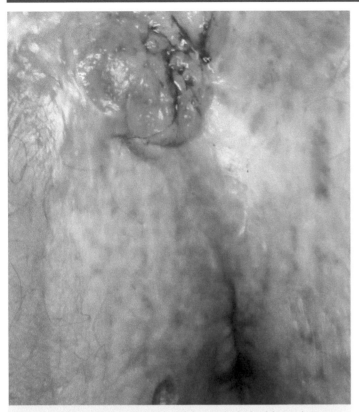

Fig. 10.2 Advanced anogenital lichen sclerosus. The leukoplakic anal margin shows an exophytic lesion and a small ulcer, both suspicious for malignancy.

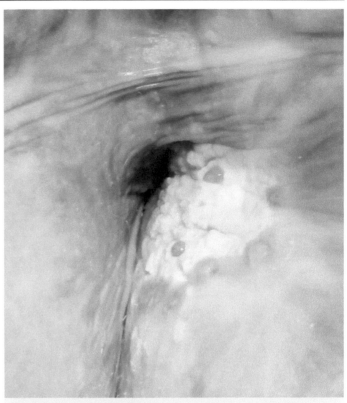

Fig. 10.3 Circumscribed leukoplakia of the anal margin in a patient with advanced anogenital lichen sclerosus. Histology showed changes similar to differentiated vulvar intraepithelial neoplasia.

leukoplakia, pigmentation, or verrucous lesions. The lesions are usually flat and solitary; 10 to 20% of patients have multiple foci (Fig. 10.5).

10.4 Diagnostic Methods for AIN

10.4.1 Colposcopy of the Anus (Anoscopy)

Anoscopy permits more precise evaluation and earlier detection of lesions than inspection with the naked eye. Perianal lesions are easily exposed by spreading the buttocks and can be visualized with a conventional colposcope. Lesions of the rectal TZ in the anal canal are visualized with an anoscope. The standard technique is to treat the perianal and anal area with 3% acetic acid for a few minutes and then insert a disposable anoscope and evaluate under magnification. The acetic acid–tissue reaction causes the dysplastic tissue to appear whitish. The squamocolumnar epithelial area is examined looking for acetowhite and for abnormal vascular changes such as punctation and mosaic patterns. Lugol's solution can also be used, and suspicious areas with AIN should appear yellow against the brownish background of the normal tissue.

The 2011 International Federation for Cervical Pathology and Colposcopy (IFCPC) terminology for anal findings includes acetowhite epithelium, punctation, atypical vessels, surface irregularities, and abnormal squamocolumnar junction as abnormal colposcopic findings (Figs. 10.6–10.8). In contrast to other sites, the terminology does not distinguish between minor and major changes.

10.4.2 Cytology

Cytology of the anal canal is done by inserting a swab or brush into the anus and rotating it to collect the cells. Patients should avoid anal intercourse for 24 hours before the examination.

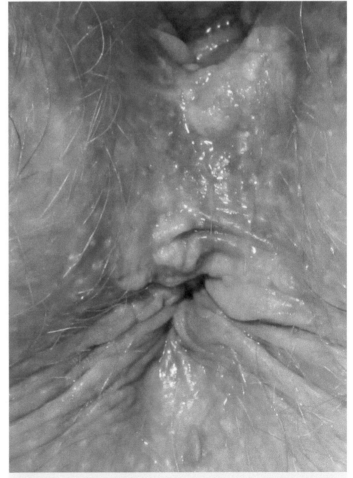

Fig. 10.4 AIN as part of multifocal HPV-associated disease. Note the perianal lesion and the lesion located at the vulva.

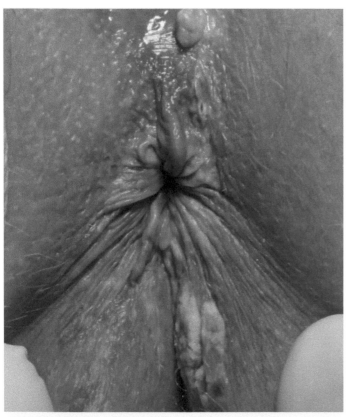

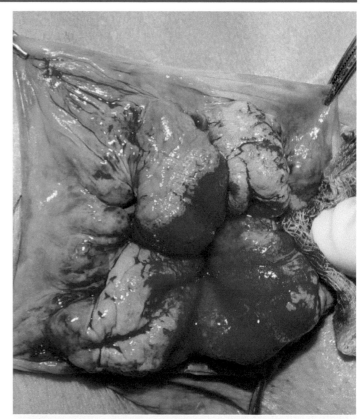

Fig. 10.5 Multiple foci of AIN. Note leukoplakia at 6 o'clock position and verrucous lesion at 12 o'clock position.

Fig. 10.7 Dense acetowhite epithelium at the anal transformation zone. (This image is provided courtesy of A. Salat.)

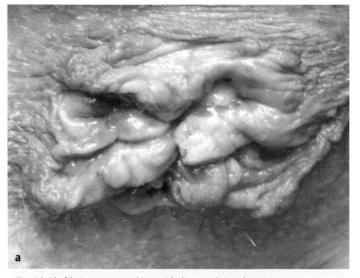

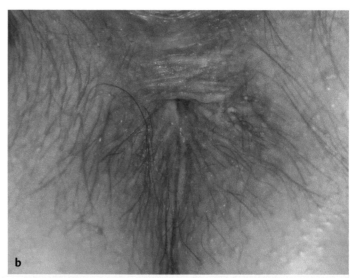

Fig. 10.6(a,b) Dense acetowhite epithelium at the anal margin.

The sensitivity of anal cytology for HG-AIN is 69 to 93% and the specificity is 32 to 59%. Keratosis may cause false-negative cytologic results. Patients who have abnormalities on cytologic testing should be referred for anoscopy with or without biopsy.

10.4.3 Biopsy

Lesions suspicious for AIN or invasive disease should undergo biopsy.

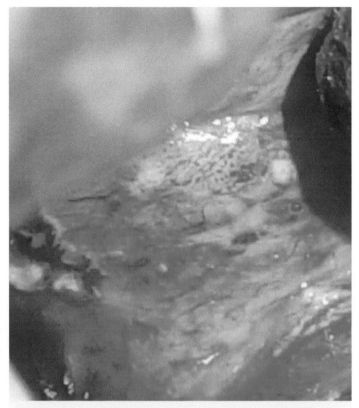

Fig. 10.8 Iodine-positive coarse punctation at the anal canal. (This image is provided courtesy of A. Salat.)

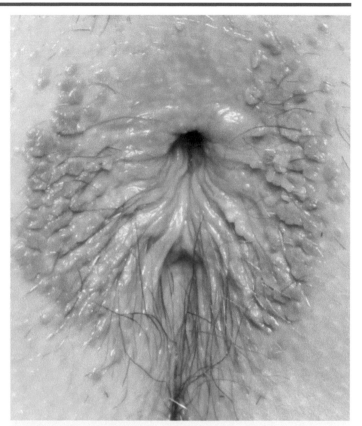

Fig. 10.9 Perianal condylomas.

10.4.4 Biomarkers

HPV testing is performed to distinguish between low-risk and high-risk infections. HPV results are helpful for triage of unclear findings and in follow-up after treatment for AIN. Staining for p16^{INK4a} may provide additional help when deciding between treatment and expectant management.

10.5 Histologic Terminology and Classification

AIN is graded histologically, much like CIN (Table 10.1). Use of the terms LG-AIN to describe mild dysplastic lesions including condylomatous changes (Fig. 10.9) and HG-AIN to describe moderate and severe dysplastic lesions helps plan appropriate management.

In 2012, the Lower Anogenital Squamous Terminology (LAST) project recommended a uniform two-tiered terminology for HPV-associated squamous disease across all anogenital tract tissues.

10.6 Management of AIN

Treatment methods for AIN are similar to those for VIN and can be divided into surgical and medical therapies. HG-AIN should be referred to specialists for treatment and follow-up.

Table 10.1 Terminology of premalignant anal and perianal squamous epithelial lesions

Classification	Synonyms
AIN, grade 1	Mild dysplasia; LG-AIN
AIN, grade 2	Moderate dysplasia; HG-AIN
AIN, grade 3	Severe dysplasia; HG-AIN; carcinoma in situ

Abbreviations: AIN, anal intraepithelial neoplasia; HG, high grade; LG, low grade.

10.6.1 Surgical Therapy

Surgical therapy consists of excision or ablation. The aim is to remove all visibly affected areas with a 3 to 5 mm margin of normal-appearing skin or mucosa (Fig. 10.10). Lesions that may be invasive and AIN involving the perianal skin with hair and glands should generally be excised and the specimens sent for careful histology. Anogenital warts and LG-AIN can be ablated with a laser to a depth of about 2 mm. Recurrences occur in 23 to 80% of treated patients.

10.6.2 Medical Therapy

A Cochrane review identified no consensus and few data from randomized trials on the optimal management of AIN. There have been

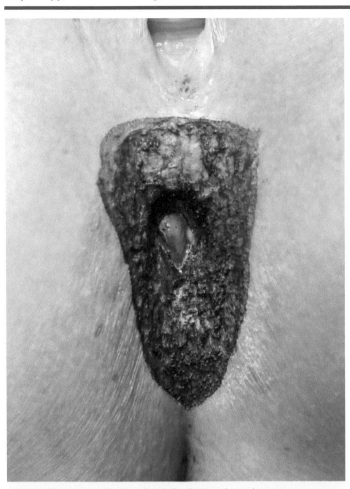

Fig. 10.10 Laser vaporization of multifocal AIN at the anal margin.

encouraging results from rails using topical imiquimod, 5-fluoro-uracil, and cidofovir for the treatment of HG-AIN. However, most of these studies have been done in men who have sex with men and thus may not apply to women. Medical treatments are frequently combined with surgical modalities, such as ablation.

Further Reading

Bornstein J, Sideri M, Tatti S, Walker P, Prendiville W, Haefner HK; Nomenclature Committee of International Federation for Cervical Pathology and Colposcopy. 2011 terminology of the vulva of the International Federation for Cervical Pathology and Colposcopy. J Low Genit Tract Dis 2012;16(3):290–295

Cachay ER, Agmas W, Mathews WC. Relative accuracy of cervical and anal cytology for detection of high grade lesions by colposcope guided biopsy: a cut-point meta-analytic comparison. PLoS ONE 2012;7(7):e38956

Edgren G, Sparén P. Risk of anogenital cancer after diagnosis of cervical intraepithelial neoplasia: a prospective population-based study. Lancet Oncol 2007;8(4):311–316

Macaya A, Muñoz-Santos C, Balaguer A, Barberà MJ. Interventions for anal canal intraepithelial neoplasia. Cochrane Database Syst Rev 2012;12:CD009244

Palefsky JM, Holly EA, Hogeboom CJ, Berry JM, Jay N, Darragh TM. Anal cytology as a screening tool for anal squamous intraepithelial lesions. J Acquir Immune Defic Syndr Hum Retrovirol 1997;14(5):415–422

Palefsky JM, Holly EA, Ralston ML, Da Costa M, Greenblatt RM. Prevalence and risk factors for anal human papillomavirus infection in human immunodeficiency virus (HIV)-positive and high-risk HIV-negative women. J Infect Dis 2001;183(3):383–391

Pandey P. Anal anatomy and normal histology. Sex Health 2012;9(6):513–516

Saleem AM, Paulus JK, Shapter AP, Baxter NN, Roberts PL, Ricciardi R. Risk of anal cancer in a cohort with human papillomavirus-related gynecologic neoplasm. Obstet Gynecol 2011;117(3):643–649

Santoso JT, Long M, Crigger M, Wan JY, Haefner HK. Anal intraepithelial neoplasia in women with genital intraepithelial neoplasia. Obstet Gynecol 2010;116(3):578–582

Scholefield JH, Harris D, Radcliffe A. Guidelines for management of anal intraepithelial neoplasia. Colorectal Dis 2011;13(Suppl 1):3–10

Simpson JA, Scholefield JH. Diagnosis and management of anal intraepithelial neoplasia and anal cancer. BMJ 2011;343:d6818

Welton ML, Lambert R, Bosman FT. Tumours of the anal canal. In: Bosman FT, Carneiro F, Hruban RH, Theise ND, eds. WHO Classification of Tumours of the Digestive System. Lyon: IARC Press; 2010

Index

Page numbers in *italics* refer to illustrations; those in **bold** refer to tables